THIS BOOK BELONGS TO:

IN CASE OF EMERGENCY CONTACT:

____

____

____

IN CASE OF EMERGENCY CONTACT:

____

____

____

IN CASE OF EMERGENCY CONTACT:

____

____

____

DEDICATION

This Diabetes Log Book is dedicated to all the children who want to track and collect data to keep their diabetes under control. Staying organized will help you share valuable information with your parents and health care providers.

You are my inspiration for producing this book and I'm honored to be a part of your record-keeping and ongoing health care.

HOW TO USE THIS BOOK

This Diabetes Log Book will help guide you by accurately recording blood glucose levels throughout the day.

Here are examples of tracking and prompts for you to fill in and write the details of your blood sugar readings throughout the day:

1. Emergency Contact Information - Fill in your important contact information.
2. Daily Log - Monday through Friday- record daily readings for blood sugar for each day.
3. Notes - A place to write additional information: snacks, carbs, exercise, and insulin doses, medications, etc.

DATE	MEALS	BEFORE	AFTER	NOTES
SUN	Breakfast			
	Lunch			
	Supper			
	Snack			
	Bedtime			

DATE	MEALS	BEFORE	AFTER	NOTES
MON	Breakfast			
	Lunch			
	Supper			
	Snack			
	Bedtime			

DATE	MEALS	BEFORE	AFTER	NOTES
TUES	Breakfast			
	Lunch			
	Supper			
	Snack			
	Bedtime			

DATE	MEALS	BEFORE	AFTER	NOTES
WED	Breakfast			
	Lunch			
	Supper			
	Snack			
	Bedtime			

DATE	MEALS	BEFORE	AFTER	NOTES
THUR	Breakfast			
	Lunch			
	Supper			
	Snack			
	Bedtime			

DATE	MEALS	BEFORE	AFTER	NOTES
FRI	Breakfast			
	Lunch			
	Supper			
	Snack			
	Bedtime			

DATE	MEALS	BEFORE	AFTER	NOTES
SAT	Breakfast			
	Lunch			
	Supper			
	Snack			
	Bedtime			

DATE	MEALS	BEFORE	AFTER	NOTES
SUN	Breakfast			
	Lunch			
	Supper			
	Snack			
	Bedtime			

DATE	MEALS	BEFORE	AFTER	NOTES
MON	Breakfast			
	Lunch			
	Supper			
	Snack			
	Bedtime			

DATE	MEALS	BEFORE	AFTER	NOTES
TUES	Breakfast			
	Lunch			
	Supper			
	Snack			
	Bedtime			

DATE	MEALS	BEFORE	AFTER	NOTES
WED	Breakfast			
	Lunch			
	Supper			
	Snack			
	Bedtime			

DATE	MEALS	BEFORE	AFTER	NOTES
THUR	Breakfast			
	Lunch			
	Supper			
	Snack			
	Bedtime			

DATE	MEALS	BEFORE	AFTER	NOTES
FRI	Breakfast			
	Lunch			
	Supper			
	Snack			
	Bedtime			

DATE	MEALS	BEFORE	AFTER	NOTES
SAT	Breakfast			
	Lunch			
	Supper			
	Snack			
	Bedtime			

DATE	MEALS	BEFORE	AFTER	NOTES
SUN	Breakfast			
	Lunch			
	Supper			
	Snack			
	Bedtime			

DATE	MEALS	BEFORE	AFTER	NOTES
MON	Breakfast			
	Lunch			
	Supper			
	Snack			
	Bedtime			

DATE	MEALS	BEFORE	AFTER	NOTES
TUES	Breakfast			
	Lunch			
	Supper			
	Snack			
	Bedtime			

DATE	MEALS	BEFORE	AFTER	NOTES
WED	Breakfast			
	Lunch			
	Supper			
	Snack			
	Bedtime			

DATE	MEALS	BEFORE	AFTER	NOTES
THUR	Breakfast			
	Lunch			
	Supper			
	Snack			
	Bedtime			

DATE	MEALS	BEFORE	AFTER	NOTES
FRI	Breakfast			
	Lunch			
	Supper			
	Snack			
	Bedtime			

DATE	MEALS	BEFORE	AFTER	NOTES
SAT	Breakfast			
	Lunch			
	Supper			
	Snack			
	Bedtime			

DATE	MEALS	BEFORE	AFTER	NOTES
SUN	Breakfast			
	Lunch			
	Supper			
	Snack			
	Bedtime			

DATE	MEALS	BEFORE	AFTER	NOTES
MON	Breakfast			
	Lunch			
	Supper			
	Snack			
	Bedtime			

DATE	MEALS	BEFORE	AFTER	NOTES
TUES	Breakfast			
	Lunch			
	Supper			
	Snack			
	Bedtime			

DATE	MEALS	BEFORE	AFTER	NOTES
WED	Breakfast			
	Lunch			
	Supper			
	Snack			
	Bedtime			

DATE	MEALS	BEFORE	AFTER	NOTES
THUR	Breakfast			
	Lunch			
	Supper			
	Snack			
	Bedtime			

DATE	MEALS	BEFORE	AFTER	NOTES
FRI	Breakfast			
	Lunch			
	Supper			
	Snack			
	Bedtime			

DATE	MEALS	BEFORE	AFTER	NOTES
SAT	Breakfast			
	Lunch			
	Supper			
	Snack			
	Bedtime			

DATE	MEALS	BEFORE	AFTER	NOTES
SUN	Breakfast			
	Lunch			
	Supper			
	Snack			
	Bedtime			

DATE	MEALS	BEFORE	AFTER	NOTES
MON	Breakfast			
	Lunch			
	Supper			
	Snack			
	Bedtime			

DATE	MEALS	BEFORE	AFTER	NOTES
TUES	Breakfast			
	Lunch			
	Supper			
	Snack			
	Bedtime			

DATE	MEALS	BEFORE	AFTER	NOTES
WED	Breakfast			
	Lunch			
	Supper			
	Snack			
	Bedtime			

DATE	MEALS	BEFORE	AFTER	NOTES
THUR	Breakfast			
	Lunch			
	Supper			
	Snack			
	Bedtime			

DATE	MEALS	BEFORE	AFTER	NOTES
FRI	Breakfast			
	Lunch			
	Supper			
	Snack			
	Bedtime			

DATE	MEALS	BEFORE	AFTER	NOTES
SAT	Breakfast			
	Lunch			
	Supper			
	Snack			
	Bedtime			

DATE	MEALS	BEFORE	AFTER	NOTES
SUN	Breakfast			
	Lunch			
	Supper			
	Snack			
	Bedtime			

DATE	MEALS	BEFORE	AFTER	NOTES
MON	Breakfast			
	Lunch			
	Supper			
	Snack			
	Bedtime			

DATE	MEALS	BEFORE	AFTER	NOTES
TUES	Breakfast			
	Lunch			
	Supper			
	Snack			
	Bedtime			

DATE	MEALS	BEFORE	AFTER	NOTES
WED	Breakfast			
	Lunch			
	Supper			
	Snack			
	Bedtime			

DATE	MEALS	BEFORE	AFTER	NOTES
THUR	Breakfast			
	Lunch			
	Supper			
	Snack			
	Bedtime			

DATE	MEALS	BEFORE	AFTER	NOTES
FRI	Breakfast			
	Lunch			
	Supper			
	Snack			
	Bedtime			

DATE	MEALS	BEFORE	AFTER	NOTES
SAT	Breakfast			
	Lunch			
	Supper			
	Snack			
	Bedtime			

DATE	MEALS	BEFORE	AFTER	NOTES
SUN	Breakfast			
	Lunch			
	Supper			
	Snack			
	Bedtime			

DATE	MEALS	BEFORE	AFTER	NOTES
MON	Breakfast			
	Lunch			
	Supper			
	Snack			
	Bedtime			

DATE	MEALS	BEFORE	AFTER	NOTES
TUES	Breakfast			
	Lunch			
	Supper			
	Snack			
	Bedtime			

DATE	MEALS	BEFORE	AFTER	NOTES
WED	Breakfast			
	Lunch			
	Supper			
	Snack			
	Bedtime			

DATE	MEALS	BEFORE	AFTER	NOTES
THUR	Breakfast			
	Lunch			
	Supper			
	Snack			
	Bedtime			

DATE	MEALS	BEFORE	AFTER	NOTES
FRI	Breakfast			
	Lunch			
	Supper			
	Snack			
	Bedtime			

DATE	MEALS	BEFORE	AFTER	NOTES
SAT	Breakfast			
	Lunch			
	Supper			
	Snack			
	Bedtime			

DATE	MEALS	BEFORE	AFTER	NOTES
SUN	Breakfast			
	Lunch			
	Supper			
	Snack			
	Bedtime			

DATE	MEALS	BEFORE	AFTER	NOTES
MON	Breakfast			
	Lunch			
	Supper			
	Snack			
	Bedtime			

DATE	MEALS	BEFORE	AFTER	NOTES
TUES	Breakfast			
	Lunch			
	Supper			
	Snack			
	Bedtime			

DATE	MEALS	BEFORE	AFTER	NOTES
WED	Breakfast			
	Lunch			
	Supper			
	Snack			
	Bedtime			

DATE	MEALS	BEFORE	AFTER	NOTES
THUR	Breakfast			
	Lunch			
	Supper			
	Snack			
	Bedtime			

DATE	MEALS	BEFORE	AFTER	NOTES
FRI	Breakfast			
	Lunch			
	Supper			
	Snack			
	Bedtime			

DATE	MEALS	BEFORE	AFTER	NOTES
SAT	Breakfast			
	Lunch			
	Supper			
	Snack			
	Bedtime			

DATE	MEALS	BEFORE	AFTER	NOTES
SUN	Breakfast			
	Lunch			
	Supper			
	Snack			
	Bedtime			

DATE	MEALS	BEFORE	AFTER	NOTES
MON	Breakfast			
	Lunch			
	Supper			
	Snack			
	Bedtime			

DATE	MEALS	BEFORE	AFTER	NOTES
TUES	Breakfast			
	Lunch			
	Supper			
	Snack			
	Bedtime			

DATE	MEALS	BEFORE	AFTER	NOTES
WED	Breakfast			
	Lunch			
	Supper			
	Snack			
	Bedtime			

DATE	MEALS	BEFORE	AFTER	NOTES
THUR	Breakfast			
	Lunch			
	Supper			
	Snack			
	Bedtime			

DATE	MEALS	BEFORE	AFTER	NOTES
FRI	Breakfast			
	Lunch			
	Supper			
	Snack			
	Bedtime			

DATE	MEALS	BEFORE	AFTER	NOTES
SAT	Breakfast			
	Lunch			
	Supper			
	Snack			
	Bedtime			

DATE	MEALS	BEFORE	AFTER	NOTES
SUN	Breakfast			
	Lunch			
	Supper			
	Snack			
	Bedtime			

DATE	MEALS	BEFORE	AFTER	NOTES
MON	Breakfast			
	Lunch			
	Supper			
	Snack			
	Bedtime			

DATE	MEALS	BEFORE	AFTER	NOTES
TUES	Breakfast			
	Lunch			
	Supper			
	Snack			
	Bedtime			

DATE	MEALS	BEFORE	AFTER	NOTES
WED	Breakfast			
	Lunch			
	Supper			
	Snack			
	Bedtime			

DATE	MEALS	BEFORE	AFTER	NOTES
THUR	Breakfast			
	Lunch			
	Supper			
	Snack			
	Bedtime			

DATE	MEALS	BEFORE	AFTER	NOTES
FRI	Breakfast			
	Lunch			
	Supper			
	Snack			
	Bedtime			

DATE	MEALS	BEFORE	AFTER	NOTES
SAT	Breakfast			
	Lunch			
	Supper			
	Snack			
	Bedtime			

DATE	MEALS	BEFORE	AFTER	NOTES
SUN	Breakfast			
	Lunch			
	Supper			
	Snack			
	Bedtime			

DATE	MEALS	BEFORE	AFTER	NOTES
MON	Breakfast			
	Lunch			
	Supper			
	Snack			
	Bedtime			

DATE	MEALS	BEFORE	AFTER	NOTES
TUES	Breakfast			
	Lunch			
	Supper			
	Snack			
	Bedtime			

DATE	MEALS	BEFORE	AFTER	NOTES
WED	Breakfast			
	Lunch			
	Supper			
	Snack			
	Bedtime			

DATE	MEALS	BEFORE	AFTER	NOTES
THUR	Breakfast			
	Lunch			
	Supper			
	Snack			
	Bedtime			

DATE	MEALS	BEFORE	AFTER	NOTES
FRI	Breakfast			
	Lunch			
	Supper			
	Snack			
	Bedtime			

DATE	MEALS	BEFORE	AFTER	NOTES
SAT	Breakfast			
	Lunch			
	Supper			
	Snack			
	Bedtime			

DATE	MEALS	BEFORE	AFTER	NOTES
SUN	Breakfast			
	Lunch			
	Supper			
	Snack			
	Bedtime			

DATE	MEALS	BEFORE	AFTER	NOTES
MON	Breakfast			
	Lunch			
	Supper			
	Snack			
	Bedtime			

DATE	MEALS	BEFORE	AFTER	NOTES
TUES	Breakfast			
	Lunch			
	Supper			
	Snack			
	Bedtime			

DATE	MEALS	BEFORE	AFTER	NOTES
WED	Breakfast			
	Lunch			
	Supper			
	Snack			
	Bedtime			

DATE	MEALS	BEFORE	AFTER	NOTES
THUR	Breakfast			
	Lunch			
	Supper			
	Snack			
	Bedtime			

DATE	MEALS	BEFORE	AFTER	NOTES
FRI	Breakfast			
	Lunch			
	Supper			
	Snack			
	Bedtime			

DATE	MEALS	BEFORE	AFTER	NOTES
SAT	Breakfast			
	Lunch			
	Supper			
	Snack			
	Bedtime			

DATE	MEALS	BEFORE	AFTER	NOTES
SUN	Breakfast			
	Lunch			
	Supper			
	Snack			
	Bedtime			

DATE	MEALS	BEFORE	AFTER	NOTES
MON	Breakfast			
	Lunch			
	Supper			
	Snack			
	Bedtime			

DATE	MEALS	BEFORE	AFTER	NOTES
TUES	Breakfast			
	Lunch			
	Supper			
	Snack			
	Bedtime			

DATE	MEALS	BEFORE	AFTER	NOTES
WED	Breakfast			
	Lunch			
	Supper			
	Snack			
	Bedtime			

DATE	MEALS	BEFORE	AFTER	NOTES
THUR	Breakfast			
	Lunch			
	Supper			
	Snack			
	Bedtime			

DATE	MEALS	BEFORE	AFTER	NOTES
FRI	Breakfast			
	Lunch			
	Supper			
	Snack			
	Bedtime			

DATE	MEALS	BEFORE	AFTER	NOTES
SAT	Breakfast			
	Lunch			
	Supper			
	Snack			
	Bedtime			

DATE	MEALS	BEFORE	AFTER	NOTES
SUN	Breakfast			
	Lunch			
	Supper			
	Snack			
	Bedtime			

DATE	MEALS	BEFORE	AFTER	NOTES
MON	Breakfast			
	Lunch			
	Supper			
	Snack			
	Bedtime			

DATE	MEALS	BEFORE	AFTER	NOTES
TUES	Breakfast			
	Lunch			
	Supper			
	Snack			
	Bedtime			

DATE	MEALS	BEFORE	AFTER	NOTES
WED	Breakfast			
	Lunch			
	Supper			
	Snack			
	Bedtime			

DATE	MEALS	BEFORE	AFTER	NOTES
THUR	Breakfast			
	Lunch			
	Supper			
	Snack			
	Bedtime			

DATE	MEALS	BEFORE	AFTER	NOTES
FRI	Breakfast			
	Lunch			
	Supper			
	Snack			
	Bedtime			

DATE	MEALS	BEFORE	AFTER	NOTES
SAT	Breakfast			
	Lunch			
	Supper			
	Snack			
	Bedtime			

DATE	MEALS	BEFORE	AFTER	NOTES
SUN	Breakfast			
	Lunch			
	Supper			
	Snack			
	Bedtime			

DATE	MEALS	BEFORE	AFTER	NOTES
MON	Breakfast			
	Lunch			
	Supper			
	Snack			
	Bedtime			

DATE	MEALS	BEFORE	AFTER	NOTES
TUES	Breakfast			
	Lunch			
	Supper			
	Snack			
	Bedtime			

DATE	MEALS	BEFORE	AFTER	NOTES
WED	Breakfast			
	Lunch			
	Supper			
	Snack			
	Bedtime			

DATE	MEALS	BEFORE	AFTER	NOTES
THUR	Breakfast			
	Lunch			
	Supper			
	Snack			
	Bedtime			

DATE	MEALS	BEFORE	AFTER	NOTES
FRI	Breakfast			
	Lunch			
	Supper			
	Snack			
	Bedtime			

DATE	MEALS	BEFORE	AFTER	NOTES
SAT	Breakfast			
	Lunch			
	Supper			
	Snack			
	Bedtime			

DATE	MEALS	BEFORE	AFTER	NOTES
SUN	Breakfast			
	Lunch			
	Supper			
	Snack			
	Bedtime			

DATE	MEALS	BEFORE	AFTER	NOTES
MON	Breakfast			
	Lunch			
	Supper			
	Snack			
	Bedtime			

DATE	MEALS	BEFORE	AFTER	NOTES
TUES	Breakfast			
	Lunch			
	Supper			
	Snack			
	Bedtime			

DATE	MEALS	BEFORE	AFTER	NOTES
WED	Breakfast			
	Lunch			
	Supper			
	Snack			
	Bedtime			

DATE	MEALS	BEFORE	AFTER	NOTES
THUR	Breakfast			
	Lunch			
	Supper			
	Snack			
	Bedtime			

DATE	MEALS	BEFORE	AFTER	NOTES
FRI	Breakfast			
	Lunch			
	Supper			
	Snack			
	Bedtime			

DATE	MEALS	BEFORE	AFTER	NOTES
SAT	Breakfast			
	Lunch			
	Supper			
	Snack			
	Bedtime			

DATE	MEALS	BEFORE	AFTER	NOTES
SUN	Breakfast			
	Lunch			
	Supper			
	Snack			
	Bedtime			

DATE	MEALS	BEFORE	AFTER	NOTES
MON	Breakfast			
	Lunch			
	Supper			
	Snack			
	Bedtime			

DATE	MEALS	BEFORE	AFTER	NOTES
TUES	Breakfast			
	Lunch			
	Supper			
	Snack			
	Bedtime			

DATE	MEALS	BEFORE	AFTER	NOTES
WED	Breakfast			
	Lunch			
	Supper			
	Snack			
	Bedtime			

DATE	MEALS	BEFORE	AFTER	NOTES
THUR	Breakfast			
	Lunch			
	Supper			
	Snack			
	Bedtime			

DATE	MEALS	BEFORE	AFTER	NOTES
FRI	Breakfast			
	Lunch			
	Supper			
	Snack			
	Bedtime			

DATE	MEALS	BEFORE	AFTER	NOTES
SAT	Breakfast			
	Lunch			
	Supper			
	Snack			
	Bedtime			

DATE	MEALS	BEFORE	AFTER	NOTES
SUN	Breakfast			
	Lunch			
	Supper			
	Snack			
	Bedtime			

DATE	MEALS	BEFORE	AFTER	NOTES
MON	Breakfast			
	Lunch			
	Supper			
	Snack			
	Bedtime			

DATE	MEALS	BEFORE	AFTER	NOTES
TUES	Breakfast			
	Lunch			
	Supper			
	Snack			
	Bedtime			

DATE	MEALS	BEFORE	AFTER	NOTES
WED	Breakfast			
	Lunch			
	Supper			
	Snack			
	Bedtime			

DATE	MEALS	BEFORE	AFTER	NOTES
THUR	Breakfast			
	Lunch			
	Supper			
	Snack			
	Bedtime			

DATE	MEALS	BEFORE	AFTER	NOTES
FRI	Breakfast			
	Lunch			
	Supper			
	Snack			
	Bedtime			

DATE	MEALS	BEFORE	AFTER	NOTES
SAT	Breakfast			
	Lunch			
	Supper			
	Snack			
	Bedtime			

DATE	MEALS	BEFORE	AFTER	NOTES
SUN	Breakfast			
	Lunch			
	Supper			
	Snack			
	Bedtime			

DATE	MEALS	BEFORE	AFTER	NOTES
MON	Breakfast			
	Lunch			
	Supper			
	Snack			
	Bedtime			

DATE	MEALS	BEFORE	AFTER	NOTES
TUES	Breakfast			
	Lunch			
	Supper			
	Snack			
	Bedtime			

DATE	MEALS	BEFORE	AFTER	NOTES
WED	Breakfast			
	Lunch			
	Supper			
	Snack			
	Bedtime			

DATE	MEALS	BEFORE	AFTER	NOTES
THUR	Breakfast			
	Lunch			
	Supper			
	Snack			
	Bedtime			

DATE	MEALS	BEFORE	AFTER	NOTES
FRI	Breakfast			
	Lunch			
	Supper			
	Snack			
	Bedtime			

DATE	MEALS	BEFORE	AFTER	NOTES
SAT	Breakfast			
	Lunch			
	Supper			
	Snack			
	Bedtime			

DATE	MEALS	BEFORE	AFTER	NOTES
SUN	Breakfast			
	Lunch			
	Supper			
	Snack			
	Bedtime			

DATE	MEALS	BEFORE	AFTER	NOTES
MON	Breakfast			
	Lunch			
	Supper			
	Snack			
	Bedtime			

DATE	MEALS	BEFORE	AFTER	NOTES
TUES	Breakfast			
	Lunch			
	Supper			
	Snack			
	Bedtime			

DATE	MEALS	BEFORE	AFTER	NOTES
WED	Breakfast			
	Lunch			
	Supper			
	Snack			
	Bedtime			

DATE	MEALS	BEFORE	AFTER	NOTES
THUR	Breakfast			
	Lunch			
	Supper			
	Snack			
	Bedtime			

DATE	MEALS	BEFORE	AFTER	NOTES
FRI	Breakfast			
	Lunch			
	Supper			
	Snack			
	Bedtime			

DATE	MEALS	BEFORE	AFTER	NOTES
SAT	Breakfast			
	Lunch			
	Supper			
	Snack			
	Bedtime			

DATE	MEALS	BEFORE	AFTER	NOTES
SUN	Breakfast			
	Lunch			
	Supper			
	Snack			
	Bedtime			

DATE	MEALS	BEFORE	AFTER	NOTES
MON	Breakfast			
	Lunch			
	Supper			
	Snack			
	Bedtime			

DATE	MEALS	BEFORE	AFTER	NOTES
TUES	Breakfast			
	Lunch			
	Supper			
	Snack			
	Bedtime			

DATE	MEALS	BEFORE	AFTER	NOTES
WED	Breakfast			
	Lunch			
	Supper			
	Snack			
	Bedtime			

DATE	MEALS	BEFORE	AFTER	NOTES
THUR	Breakfast			
	Lunch			
	Supper			
	Snack			
	Bedtime			

DATE	MEALS	BEFORE	AFTER	NOTES
FRI	Breakfast			
	Lunch			
	Supper			
	Snack			
	Bedtime			

DATE	MEALS	BEFORE	AFTER	NOTES
SAT	Breakfast			
	Lunch			
	Supper			
	Snack			
	Bedtime			

DATE	MEALS	BEFORE	AFTER	NOTES
SUN	Breakfast			
	Lunch			
	Supper			
	Snack			
	Bedtime			

DATE	MEALS	BEFORE	AFTER	NOTES
MON	Breakfast			
	Lunch			
	Supper			
	Snack			
	Bedtime			

DATE	MEALS	BEFORE	AFTER	NOTES
TUES	Breakfast			
	Lunch			
	Supper			
	Snack			
	Bedtime			

DATE	MEALS	BEFORE	AFTER	NOTES
WED	Breakfast			
	Lunch			
	Supper			
	Snack			
	Bedtime			

DATE	MEALS	BEFORE	AFTER	NOTES
THUR	Breakfast			
	Lunch			
	Supper			
	Snack			
	Bedtime			

DATE	MEALS	BEFORE	AFTER	NOTES
FRI	Breakfast			
	Lunch			
	Supper			
	Snack			
	Bedtime			

DATE	MEALS	BEFORE	AFTER	NOTES
SAT	Breakfast			
	Lunch			
	Supper			
	Snack			
	Bedtime			

DATE	MEALS	BEFORE	AFTER	NOTES
SUN	Breakfast			
	Lunch			
	Supper			
	Snack			
	Bedtime			

DATE	MEALS	BEFORE	AFTER	NOTES
MON	Breakfast			
	Lunch			
	Supper			
	Snack			
	Bedtime			

DATE	MEALS	BEFORE	AFTER	NOTES
TUES	Breakfast			
	Lunch			
	Supper			
	Snack			
	Bedtime			

DATE	MEALS	BEFORE	AFTER	NOTES
WED	Breakfast			
	Lunch			
	Supper			
	Snack			
	Bedtime			

DATE	MEALS	BEFORE	AFTER	NOTES
THUR	Breakfast			
	Lunch			
	Supper			
	Snack			
	Bedtime			

DATE	MEALS	BEFORE	AFTER	NOTES
FRI	Breakfast			
	Lunch			
	Supper			
	Snack			
	Bedtime			

DATE	MEALS	BEFORE	AFTER	NOTES
SAT	Breakfast			
	Lunch			
	Supper			
	Snack			
	Bedtime			

DATE	MEALS	BEFORE	AFTER	NOTES
SUN	Breakfast			
	Lunch			
	Supper			
	Snack			
	Bedtime			

DATE	MEALS	BEFORE	AFTER	NOTES
MON	Breakfast			
	Lunch			
	Supper			
	Snack			
	Bedtime			

DATE	MEALS	BEFORE	AFTER	NOTES
TUES	Breakfast			
	Lunch			
	Supper			
	Snack			
	Bedtime			

DATE	MEALS	BEFORE	AFTER	NOTES
WED	Breakfast			
	Lunch			
	Supper			
	Snack			
	Bedtime			

DATE	MEALS	BEFORE	AFTER	NOTES
THUR	Breakfast			
	Lunch			
	Supper			
	Snack			
	Bedtime			

DATE	MEALS	BEFORE	AFTER	NOTES
FRI	Breakfast			
	Lunch			
	Supper			
	Snack			
	Bedtime			

DATE	MEALS	BEFORE	AFTER	NOTES
SAT	Breakfast			
	Lunch			
	Supper			
	Snack			
	Bedtime			

DATE	MEALS	BEFORE	AFTER	NOTES
SUN	Breakfast			
	Lunch			
	Supper			
	Snack			
	Bedtime			

DATE	MEALS	BEFORE	AFTER	NOTES
MON	Breakfast			
	Lunch			
	Supper			
	Snack			
	Bedtime			

DATE	MEALS	BEFORE	AFTER	NOTES
TUES	Breakfast			
	Lunch			
	Supper			
	Snack			
	Bedtime			

DATE	MEALS	BEFORE	AFTER	NOTES
WED	Breakfast			
	Lunch			
	Supper			
	Snack			
	Bedtime			

DATE	MEALS	BEFORE	AFTER	NOTES
THUR	Breakfast			
	Lunch			
	Supper			
	Snack			
	Bedtime			

DATE	MEALS	BEFORE	AFTER	NOTES
FRI	Breakfast			
	Lunch			
	Supper			
	Snack			
	Bedtime			

DATE	MEALS	BEFORE	AFTER	NOTES
SAT	Breakfast			
	Lunch			
	Supper			
	Snack			
	Bedtime			

DATE	MEALS	BEFORE	AFTER	NOTES
SUN	Breakfast			
	Lunch			
	Supper			
	Snack			
	Bedtime			

DATE	MEALS	BEFORE	AFTER	NOTES
MON	Breakfast			
	Lunch			
	Supper			
	Snack			
	Bedtime			

DATE	MEALS	BEFORE	AFTER	NOTES
TUES	Breakfast			
	Lunch			
	Supper			
	Snack			
	Bedtime			

DATE	MEALS	BEFORE	AFTER	NOTES
WED	Breakfast			
	Lunch			
	Supper			
	Snack			
	Bedtime			

DATE	MEALS	BEFORE	AFTER	NOTES
THUR	Breakfast			
	Lunch			
	Supper			
	Snack			
	Bedtime			

DATE	MEALS	BEFORE	AFTER	NOTES
FRI	Breakfast			
	Lunch			
	Supper			
	Snack			
	Bedtime			

DATE	MEALS	BEFORE	AFTER	NOTES
SAT	Breakfast			
	Lunch			
	Supper			
	Snack			
	Bedtime			

DATE	MEALS	BEFORE	AFTER	NOTES
SUN	Breakfast			
	Lunch			
	Supper			
	Snack			
	Bedtime			

DATE	MEALS	BEFORE	AFTER	NOTES
MON	Breakfast			
	Lunch			
	Supper			
	Snack			
	Bedtime			

DATE	MEALS	BEFORE	AFTER	NOTES
TUES	Breakfast			
	Lunch			
	Supper			
	Snack			
	Bedtime			

DATE	MEALS	BEFORE	AFTER	NOTES
WED	Breakfast			
	Lunch			
	Supper			
	Snack			
	Bedtime			

DATE	MEALS	BEFORE	AFTER	NOTES
THUR	Breakfast			
	Lunch			
	Supper			
	Snack			
	Bedtime			

DATE	MEALS	BEFORE	AFTER	NOTES
FRI	Breakfast			
	Lunch			
	Supper			
	Snack			
	Bedtime			

DATE	MEALS	BEFORE	AFTER	NOTES
SAT	Breakfast			
	Lunch			
	Supper			
	Snack			
	Bedtime			

DATE	MEALS	BEFORE	AFTER	NOTES
SUN	Breakfast			
	Lunch			
	Supper			
	Snack			
	Bedtime			

DATE	MEALS	BEFORE	AFTER	NOTES
MON	Breakfast			
	Lunch			
	Supper			
	Snack			
	Bedtime			

DATE	MEALS	BEFORE	AFTER	NOTES
TUES	Breakfast			
	Lunch			
	Supper			
	Snack			
	Bedtime			

DATE	MEALS	BEFORE	AFTER	NOTES
WED	Breakfast			
	Lunch			
	Supper			
	Snack			
	Bedtime			

DATE	MEALS	BEFORE	AFTER	NOTES
THUR	Breakfast			
	Lunch			
	Supper			
	Snack			
	Bedtime			

DATE	MEALS	BEFORE	AFTER	NOTES
FRI	Breakfast			
	Lunch			
	Supper			
	Snack			
	Bedtime			

DATE	MEALS	BEFORE	AFTER	NOTES
SAT	Breakfast			
	Lunch			
	Supper			
	Snack			
	Bedtime			

DATE	MEALS	BEFORE	AFTER	NOTES
SUN	Breakfast			
	Lunch			
	Supper			
	Snack			
	Bedtime			

DATE	MEALS	BEFORE	AFTER	NOTES
MON	Breakfast			
	Lunch			
	Supper			
	Snack			
	Bedtime			

DATE	MEALS	BEFORE	AFTER	NOTES
TUES	Breakfast			
	Lunch			
	Supper			
	Snack			
	Bedtime			

DATE	MEALS	BEFORE	AFTER	NOTES
WED	Breakfast			
	Lunch			
	Supper			
	Snack			
	Bedtime			

DATE	MEALS	BEFORE	AFTER	NOTES
THUR	Breakfast			
	Lunch			
	Supper			
	Snack			
	Bedtime			

DATE	MEALS	BEFORE	AFTER	NOTES
FRI	Breakfast			
	Lunch			
	Supper			
	Snack			
	Bedtime			

DATE	MEALS	BEFORE	AFTER	NOTES
SAT	Breakfast			
	Lunch			
	Supper			
	Snack			
	Bedtime			

DATE	MEALS	BEFORE	AFTER	NOTES
SUN	Breakfast			
	Lunch			
	Supper			
	Snack			
	Bedtime			

DATE	MEALS	BEFORE	AFTER	NOTES
MON	Breakfast			
	Lunch			
	Supper			
	Snack			
	Bedtime			

DATE	MEALS	BEFORE	AFTER	NOTES
TUES	Breakfast			
	Lunch			
	Supper			
	Snack			
	Bedtime			

DATE	MEALS	BEFORE	AFTER	NOTES
WED	Breakfast			
	Lunch			
	Supper			
	Snack			
	Bedtime			

DATE	MEALS	BEFORE	AFTER	NOTES
THUR	Breakfast			
	Lunch			
	Supper			
	Snack			
	Bedtime			

DATE	MEALS	BEFORE	AFTER	NOTES
FRI	Breakfast			
	Lunch			
	Supper			
	Snack			
	Bedtime			

DATE	MEALS	BEFORE	AFTER	NOTES
SAT	Breakfast			
	Lunch			
	Supper			
	Snack			
	Bedtime			

DATE	MEALS	BEFORE	AFTER	NOTES
SUN	Breakfast			
	Lunch			
	Supper			
	Snack			
	Bedtime			

DATE	MEALS	BEFORE	AFTER	NOTES
MON	Breakfast			
	Lunch			
	Supper			
	Snack			
	Bedtime			

DATE	MEALS	BEFORE	AFTER	NOTES
TUES	Breakfast			
	Lunch			
	Supper			
	Snack			
	Bedtime			

DATE	MEALS	BEFORE	AFTER	NOTES
WED	Breakfast			
	Lunch			
	Supper			
	Snack			
	Bedtime			

DATE	MEALS	BEFORE	AFTER	NOTES
THUR	Breakfast			
	Lunch			
	Supper			
	Snack			
	Bedtime			

DATE	MEALS	BEFORE	AFTER	NOTES
FRI	Breakfast			
	Lunch			
	Supper			
	Snack			
	Bedtime			

DATE	MEALS	BEFORE	AFTER	NOTES
SAT	Breakfast			
	Lunch			
	Supper			
	Snack			
	Bedtime			

DATE	MEALS	BEFORE	AFTER	NOTES
SUN	Breakfast			
	Lunch			
	Supper			
	Snack			
	Bedtime			

DATE	MEALS	BEFORE	AFTER	NOTES
MON	Breakfast			
	Lunch			
	Supper			
	Snack			
	Bedtime			

DATE	MEALS	BEFORE	AFTER	NOTES
TUES	Breakfast			
	Lunch			
	Supper			
	Snack			
	Bedtime			

DATE	MEALS	BEFORE	AFTER	NOTES
WED	Breakfast			
	Lunch			
	Supper			
	Snack			
	Bedtime			

DATE	MEALS	BEFORE	AFTER	NOTES
THUR	Breakfast			
	Lunch			
	Supper			
	Snack			
	Bedtime			

DATE	MEALS	BEFORE	AFTER	NOTES
FRI	Breakfast			
	Lunch			
	Supper			
	Snack			
	Bedtime			

DATE	MEALS	BEFORE	AFTER	NOTES
SAT	Breakfast			
	Lunch			
	Supper			
	Snack			
	Bedtime			

DATE	MEALS	BEFORE	AFTER	NOTES
SUN	Breakfast			
	Lunch			
	Supper			
	Snack			
	Bedtime			

DATE	MEALS	BEFORE	AFTER	NOTES
MON	Breakfast			
	Lunch			
	Supper			
	Snack			
	Bedtime			

DATE	MEALS	BEFORE	AFTER	NOTES
TUES	Breakfast			
	Lunch			
	Supper			
	Snack			
	Bedtime			

DATE	MEALS	BEFORE	AFTER	NOTES
WED	Breakfast			
	Lunch			
	Supper			
	Snack			
	Bedtime			

DATE	MEALS	BEFORE	AFTER	NOTES
THUR	Breakfast			
	Lunch			
	Supper			
	Snack			
	Bedtime			

DATE	MEALS	BEFORE	AFTER	NOTES
FRI	Breakfast			
	Lunch			
	Supper			
	Snack			
	Bedtime			

DATE	MEALS	BEFORE	AFTER	NOTES
SAT	Breakfast			
	Lunch			
	Supper			
	Snack			
	Bedtime			

DATE	MEALS	BEFORE	AFTER	NOTES
SUN	Breakfast			
	Lunch			
	Supper			
	Snack			
	Bedtime			

DATE	MEALS	BEFORE	AFTER	NOTES
MON	Breakfast			
	Lunch			
	Supper			
	Snack			
	Bedtime			

DATE	MEALS	BEFORE	AFTER	NOTES
TUES	Breakfast			
	Lunch			
	Supper			
	Snack			
	Bedtime			

DATE	MEALS	BEFORE	AFTER	NOTES
WED	Breakfast			
	Lunch			
	Supper			
	Snack			
	Bedtime			

DATE	MEALS	BEFORE	AFTER	NOTES
THUR	Breakfast			
	Lunch			
	Supper			
	Snack			
	Bedtime			

DATE	MEALS	BEFORE	AFTER	NOTES
FRI	Breakfast			
	Lunch			
	Supper			
	Snack			
	Bedtime			

DATE	MEALS	BEFORE	AFTER	NOTES
SAT	Breakfast			
	Lunch			
	Supper			
	Snack			
	Bedtime			

DATE	MEALS	BEFORE	AFTER	NOTES
SUN	Breakfast			
	Lunch			
	Supper			
	Snack			
	Bedtime			

DATE	MEALS	BEFORE	AFTER	NOTES
MON	Breakfast			
	Lunch			
	Supper			
	Snack			
	Bedtime			

DATE	MEALS	BEFORE	AFTER	NOTES
TUES	Breakfast			
	Lunch			
	Supper			
	Snack			
	Bedtime			

DATE	MEALS	BEFORE	AFTER	NOTES
WED	Breakfast			
	Lunch			
	Supper			
	Snack			
	Bedtime			

DATE	MEALS	BEFORE	AFTER	NOTES
THUR	Breakfast			
	Lunch			
	Supper			
	Snack			
	Bedtime			

DATE	MEALS	BEFORE	AFTER	NOTES
FRI	Breakfast			
	Lunch			
	Supper			
	Snack			
	Bedtime			

DATE	MEALS	BEFORE	AFTER	NOTES
SAT	Breakfast			
	Lunch			
	Supper			
	Snack			
	Bedtime			

DATE	MEALS	BEFORE	AFTER	NOTES
SUN	Breakfast			
	Lunch			
	Supper			
	Snack			
	Bedtime			

DATE	MEALS	BEFORE	AFTER	NOTES
MON	Breakfast			
	Lunch			
	Supper			
	Snack			
	Bedtime			

DATE	MEALS	BEFORE	AFTER	NOTES
TUES	Breakfast			
	Lunch			
	Supper			
	Snack			
	Bedtime			

DATE	MEALS	BEFORE	AFTER	NOTES
WED	Breakfast			
	Lunch			
	Supper			
	Snack			
	Bedtime			

DATE	MEALS	BEFORE	AFTER	NOTES
THUR	Breakfast			
	Lunch			
	Supper			
	Snack			
	Bedtime			

DATE	MEALS	BEFORE	AFTER	NOTES
FRI	Breakfast			
	Lunch			
	Supper			
	Snack			
	Bedtime			

DATE	MEALS	BEFORE	AFTER	NOTES
SAT	Breakfast			
	Lunch			
	Supper			
	Snack			
	Bedtime			

DATE	MEALS	BEFORE	AFTER	NOTES
SUN	Breakfast			
	Lunch			
	Supper			
	Snack			
	Bedtime			

DATE	MEALS	BEFORE	AFTER	NOTES
MON	Breakfast			
	Lunch			
	Supper			
	Snack			
	Bedtime			

DATE	MEALS	BEFORE	AFTER	NOTES
TUES	Breakfast			
	Lunch			
	Supper			
	Snack			
	Bedtime			

DATE	MEALS	BEFORE	AFTER	NOTES
WED	Breakfast			
	Lunch			
	Supper			
	Snack			
	Bedtime			

DATE	MEALS	BEFORE	AFTER	NOTES
THUR	Breakfast			
	Lunch			
	Supper			
	Snack			
	Bedtime			

DATE	MEALS	BEFORE	AFTER	NOTES
FRI	Breakfast			
	Lunch			
	Supper			
	Snack			
	Bedtime			

DATE	MEALS	BEFORE	AFTER	NOTES
SAT	Breakfast			
	Lunch			
	Supper			
	Snack			
	Bedtime			

DATE	MEALS	BEFORE	AFTER	NOTES
SUN	Breakfast			
	Lunch			
	Supper			
	Snack			
	Bedtime			

DATE	MEALS	BEFORE	AFTER	NOTES
MON	Breakfast			
	Lunch			
	Supper			
	Snack			
	Bedtime			

DATE	MEALS	BEFORE	AFTER	NOTES
TUES	Breakfast			
	Lunch			
	Supper			
	Snack			
	Bedtime			

DATE	MEALS	BEFORE	AFTER	NOTES
WED	Breakfast			
	Lunch			
	Supper			
	Snack			
	Bedtime			

DATE	MEALS	BEFORE	AFTER	NOTES
THUR	Breakfast			
	Lunch			
	Supper			
	Snack			
	Bedtime			

DATE	MEALS	BEFORE	AFTER	NOTES
FRI	Breakfast			
	Lunch			
	Supper			
	Snack			
	Bedtime			

DATE	MEALS	BEFORE	AFTER	NOTES
SAT	Breakfast			
	Lunch			
	Supper			
	Snack			
	Bedtime			

DATE	MEALS	BEFORE	AFTER	NOTES
SUN	Breakfast			
	Lunch			
	Supper			
	Snack			
	Bedtime			

DATE	MEALS	BEFORE	AFTER	NOTES
MON	Breakfast			
	Lunch			
	Supper			
	Snack			
	Bedtime			

DATE	MEALS	BEFORE	AFTER	NOTES
TUES	Breakfast			
	Lunch			
	Supper			
	Snack			
	Bedtime			

DATE	MEALS	BEFORE	AFTER	NOTES
WED	Breakfast			
	Lunch			
	Supper			
	Snack			
	Bedtime			

DATE	MEALS	BEFORE	AFTER	NOTES
THUR	Breakfast			
	Lunch			
	Supper			
	Snack			
	Bedtime			

DATE	MEALS	BEFORE	AFTER	NOTES
FRI	Breakfast			
	Lunch			
	Supper			
	Snack			
	Bedtime			

DATE	MEALS	BEFORE	AFTER	NOTES
SAT	Breakfast			
	Lunch			
	Supper			
	Snack			
	Bedtime			

DATE	MEALS	BEFORE	AFTER	NOTES
SUN	Breakfast			
	Lunch			
	Supper			
	Snack			
	Bedtime			

DATE	MEALS	BEFORE	AFTER	NOTES
MON	Breakfast			
	Lunch			
	Supper			
	Snack			
	Bedtime			

DATE	MEALS	BEFORE	AFTER	NOTES
TUES	Breakfast			
	Lunch			
	Supper			
	Snack			
	Bedtime			

DATE	MEALS	BEFORE	AFTER	NOTES
WED	Breakfast			
	Lunch			
	Supper			
	Snack			
	Bedtime			

DATE	MEALS	BEFORE	AFTER	NOTES
THUR	Breakfast			
	Lunch			
	Supper			
	Snack			
	Bedtime			

DATE	MEALS	BEFORE	AFTER	NOTES
FRI	Breakfast			
	Lunch			
	Supper			
	Snack			
	Bedtime			

DATE	MEALS	BEFORE	AFTER	NOTES
SAT	Breakfast			
	Lunch			
	Supper			
	Snack			
	Bedtime			

DATE	MEALS	BEFORE	AFTER	NOTES
SUN	Breakfast			
	Lunch			
	Supper			
	Snack			
	Bedtime			

DATE	MEALS	BEFORE	AFTER	NOTES
MON	Breakfast			
	Lunch			
	Supper			
	Snack			
	Bedtime			

DATE	MEALS	BEFORE	AFTER	NOTES
TUES	Breakfast			
	Lunch			
	Supper			
	Snack			
	Bedtime			

DATE	MEALS	BEFORE	AFTER	NOTES
WED	Breakfast			
	Lunch			
	Supper			
	Snack			
	Bedtime			

DATE	MEALS	BEFORE	AFTER	NOTES
THUR	Breakfast			
	Lunch			
	Supper			
	Snack			
	Bedtime			

DATE	MEALS	BEFORE	AFTER	NOTES
FRI	Breakfast			
	Lunch			
	Supper			
	Snack			
	Bedtime			

DATE	MEALS	BEFORE	AFTER	NOTES
SAT	Breakfast			
	Lunch			
	Supper			
	Snack			
	Bedtime			

DATE	MEALS	BEFORE	AFTER	NOTES
SUN	Breakfast			
	Lunch			
	Supper			
	Snack			
	Bedtime			

DATE	MEALS	BEFORE	AFTER	NOTES
MON	Breakfast			
	Lunch			
	Supper			
	Snack			
	Bedtime			

DATE	MEALS	BEFORE	AFTER	NOTES
TUES	Breakfast			
	Lunch			
	Supper			
	Snack			
	Bedtime			

DATE	MEALS	BEFORE	AFTER	NOTES
WED	Breakfast			
	Lunch			
	Supper			
	Snack			
	Bedtime			

DATE	MEALS	BEFORE	AFTER	NOTES
THUR	Breakfast			
	Lunch			
	Supper			
	Snack			
	Bedtime			

DATE	MEALS	BEFORE	AFTER	NOTES
FRI	Breakfast			
	Lunch			
	Supper			
	Snack			
	Bedtime			

DATE	MEALS	BEFORE	AFTER	NOTES
SAT	Breakfast			
	Lunch			
	Supper			
	Snack			
	Bedtime			

DATE	MEALS	BEFORE	AFTER	NOTES
SUN	Breakfast			
	Lunch			
	Supper			
	Snack			
	Bedtime			

DATE	MEALS	BEFORE	AFTER	NOTES
MON	Breakfast			
	Lunch			
	Supper			
	Snack			
	Bedtime			

DATE	MEALS	BEFORE	AFTER	NOTES
TUES	Breakfast			
	Lunch			
	Supper			
	Snack			
	Bedtime			

DATE	MEALS	BEFORE	AFTER	NOTES
WED	Breakfast			
	Lunch			
	Supper			
	Snack			
	Bedtime			

DATE	MEALS	BEFORE	AFTER	NOTES
THUR	Breakfast			
	Lunch			
	Supper			
	Snack			
	Bedtime			

DATE	MEALS	BEFORE	AFTER	NOTES
FRI	Breakfast			
	Lunch			
	Supper			
	Snack			
	Bedtime			

DATE	MEALS	BEFORE	AFTER	NOTES
SAT	Breakfast			
	Lunch			
	Supper			
	Snack			
	Bedtime			

DATE	MEALS	BEFORE	AFTER	NOTES
SUN	Breakfast			
	Lunch			
	Supper			
	Snack			
	Bedtime			

DATE	MEALS	BEFORE	AFTER	NOTES
MON	Breakfast			
	Lunch			
	Supper			
	Snack			
	Bedtime			

DATE	MEALS	BEFORE	AFTER	NOTES
TUES	Breakfast			
	Lunch			
	Supper			
	Snack			
	Bedtime			

DATE	MEALS	BEFORE	AFTER	NOTES
WED	Breakfast			
	Lunch			
	Supper			
	Snack			
	Bedtime			

DATE	MEALS	BEFORE	AFTER	NOTES
THUR	Breakfast			
	Lunch			
	Supper			
	Snack			
	Bedtime			

DATE	MEALS	BEFORE	AFTER	NOTES
FRI	Breakfast			
	Lunch			
	Supper			
	Snack			
	Bedtime			

DATE	MEALS	BEFORE	AFTER	NOTES
SAT	Breakfast			
	Lunch			
	Supper			
	Snack			
	Bedtime			

DATE	MEALS	BEFORE	AFTER	NOTES
SUN	Breakfast			
	Lunch			
	Supper			
	Snack			
	Bedtime			

DATE	MEALS	BEFORE	AFTER	NOTES
MON	Breakfast			
	Lunch			
	Supper			
	Snack			
	Bedtime			

DATE	MEALS	BEFORE	AFTER	NOTES
TUES	Breakfast			
	Lunch			
	Supper			
	Snack			
	Bedtime			

DATE	MEALS	BEFORE	AFTER	NOTES
WED	Breakfast			
	Lunch			
	Supper			
	Snack			
	Bedtime			

DATE	MEALS	BEFORE	AFTER	NOTES
THUR	Breakfast			
	Lunch			
	Supper			
	Snack			
	Bedtime			

DATE	MEALS	BEFORE	AFTER	NOTES
FRI	Breakfast			
	Lunch			
	Supper			
	Snack			
	Bedtime			

DATE	MEALS	BEFORE	AFTER	NOTES
SAT	Breakfast			
	Lunch			
	Supper			
	Snack			
	Bedtime			

DATE	MEALS	BEFORE	AFTER	NOTES
SUN	Breakfast			
	Lunch			
	Supper			
	Snack			
	Bedtime			

DATE	MEALS	BEFORE	AFTER	NOTES
MON	Breakfast			
	Lunch			
	Supper			
	Snack			
	Bedtime			

DATE	MEALS	BEFORE	AFTER	NOTES
TUES	Breakfast			
	Lunch			
	Supper			
	Snack			
	Bedtime			

DATE	MEALS	BEFORE	AFTER	NOTES
WED	Breakfast			
	Lunch			
	Supper			
	Snack			
	Bedtime			

DATE	MEALS	BEFORE	AFTER	NOTES
THUR	Breakfast			
	Lunch			
	Supper			
	Snack			
	Bedtime			

DATE	MEALS	BEFORE	AFTER	NOTES
FRI	Breakfast			
	Lunch			
	Supper			
	Snack			
	Bedtime			

DATE	MEALS	BEFORE	AFTER	NOTES
SAT	Breakfast			
	Lunch			
	Supper			
	Snack			
	Bedtime			

DATE	MEALS	BEFORE	AFTER	NOTES
SUN	Breakfast			
	Lunch			
	Supper			
	Snack			
	Bedtime			

DATE	MEALS	BEFORE	AFTER	NOTES
MON	Breakfast			
	Lunch			
	Supper			
	Snack			
	Bedtime			

DATE	MEALS	BEFORE	AFTER	NOTES
TUES	Breakfast			
	Lunch			
	Supper			
	Snack			
	Bedtime			

DATE	MEALS	BEFORE	AFTER	NOTES
WED	Breakfast			
	Lunch			
	Supper			
	Snack			
	Bedtime			

DATE	MEALS	BEFORE	AFTER	NOTES
THUR	Breakfast			
	Lunch			
	Supper			
	Snack			
	Bedtime			

DATE	MEALS	BEFORE	AFTER	NOTES
FRI	Breakfast			
	Lunch			
	Supper			
	Snack			
	Bedtime			

DATE	MEALS	BEFORE	AFTER	NOTES
SAT	Breakfast			
	Lunch			
	Supper			
	Snack			
	Bedtime			

DATE	MEALS	BEFORE	AFTER	NOTES
SUN	Breakfast			
	Lunch			
	Supper			
	Snack			
	Bedtime			

DATE	MEALS	BEFORE	AFTER	NOTES
MON	Breakfast			
	Lunch			
	Supper			
	Snack			
	Bedtime			

DATE	MEALS	BEFORE	AFTER	NOTES
TUES	Breakfast			
	Lunch			
	Supper			
	Snack			
	Bedtime			

DATE	MEALS	BEFORE	AFTER	NOTES
WED	Breakfast			
	Lunch			
	Supper			
	Snack			
	Bedtime			

DATE	MEALS	BEFORE	AFTER	NOTES
THUR	Breakfast			
	Lunch			
	Supper			
	Snack			
	Bedtime			

DATE	MEALS	BEFORE	AFTER	NOTES
FRI	Breakfast			
	Lunch			
	Supper			
	Snack			
	Bedtime			

DATE	MEALS	BEFORE	AFTER	NOTES
SAT	Breakfast			
	Lunch			
	Supper			
	Snack			
	Bedtime			

DATE	MEALS	BEFORE	AFTER	NOTES
SUN	Breakfast			
	Lunch			
	Supper			
	Snack			
	Bedtime			

DATE	MEALS	BEFORE	AFTER	NOTES
MON	Breakfast			
	Lunch			
	Supper			
	Snack			
	Bedtime			

DATE	MEALS	BEFORE	AFTER	NOTES
TUES	Breakfast			
	Lunch			
	Supper			
	Snack			
	Bedtime			

DATE	MEALS	BEFORE	AFTER	NOTES
WED	Breakfast			
	Lunch			
	Supper			
	Snack			
	Bedtime			

DATE	MEALS	BEFORE	AFTER	NOTES
THUR	Breakfast			
	Lunch			
	Supper			
	Snack			
	Bedtime			

DATE	MEALS	BEFORE	AFTER	NOTES
FRI	Breakfast			
	Lunch			
	Supper			
	Snack			
	Bedtime			

DATE	MEALS	BEFORE	AFTER	NOTES
SAT	Breakfast			
	Lunch			
	Supper			
	Snack			
	Bedtime			

DATE	MEALS	BEFORE	AFTER	NOTES
SUN	Breakfast			
	Lunch			
	Supper			
	Snack			
	Bedtime			

DATE	MEALS	BEFORE	AFTER	NOTES
MON	Breakfast			
	Lunch			
	Supper			
	Snack			
	Bedtime			

DATE	MEALS	BEFORE	AFTER	NOTES
TUES	Breakfast			
	Lunch			
	Supper			
	Snack			
	Bedtime			

DATE	MEALS	BEFORE	AFTER	NOTES
WED	Breakfast			
	Lunch			
	Supper			
	Snack			
	Bedtime			

DATE	MEALS	BEFORE	AFTER	NOTES
THUR	Breakfast			
	Lunch			
	Supper			
	Snack			
	Bedtime			

DATE	MEALS	BEFORE	AFTER	NOTES
FRI	Breakfast			
	Lunch			
	Supper			
	Snack			
	Bedtime			

DATE	MEALS	BEFORE	AFTER	NOTES
SAT	Breakfast			
	Lunch			
	Supper			
	Snack			
	Bedtime			

DATE	MEALS	BEFORE	AFTER	NOTES
SUN	Breakfast			
	Lunch			
	Supper			
	Snack			
	Bedtime			

DATE	MEALS	BEFORE	AFTER	NOTES
MON	Breakfast			
	Lunch			
	Supper			
	Snack			
	Bedtime			

DATE	MEALS	BEFORE	AFTER	NOTES
TUES	Breakfast			
	Lunch			
	Supper			
	Snack			
	Bedtime			

DATE	MEALS	BEFORE	AFTER	NOTES
WED	Breakfast			
	Lunch			
	Supper			
	Snack			
	Bedtime			

DATE	MEALS	BEFORE	AFTER	NOTES
THUR	Breakfast			
	Lunch			
	Supper			
	Snack			
	Bedtime			

DATE	MEALS	BEFORE	AFTER	NOTES
FRI	Breakfast			
	Lunch			
	Supper			
	Snack			
	Bedtime			

DATE	MEALS	BEFORE	AFTER	NOTES
SAT	Breakfast			
	Lunch			
	Supper			
	Snack			
	Bedtime			

DATE	MEALS	BEFORE	AFTER	NOTES
SUN	Breakfast			
	Lunch			
	Supper			
	Snack			
	Bedtime			

DATE	MEALS	BEFORE	AFTER	NOTES
MON	Breakfast			
	Lunch			
	Supper			
	Snack			
	Bedtime			

DATE	MEALS	BEFORE	AFTER	NOTES
TUES	Breakfast			
	Lunch			
	Supper			
	Snack			
	Bedtime			

DATE	MEALS	BEFORE	AFTER	NOTES
WED	Breakfast			
	Lunch			
	Supper			
	Snack			
	Bedtime			

DATE	MEALS	BEFORE	AFTER	NOTES
THUR	Breakfast			
	Lunch			
	Supper			
	Snack			
	Bedtime			

DATE	MEALS	BEFORE	AFTER	NOTES
FRI	Breakfast			
	Lunch			
	Supper			
	Snack			
	Bedtime			

DATE	MEALS	BEFORE	AFTER	NOTES
SAT	Breakfast			
	Lunch			
	Supper			
	Snack			
	Bedtime			

DATE	MEALS	BEFORE	AFTER	NOTES
SUN	Breakfast			
	Lunch			
	Supper			
	Snack			
	Bedtime			

DATE	MEALS	BEFORE	AFTER	NOTES
MON	Breakfast			
	Lunch			
	Supper			
	Snack			
	Bedtime			

DATE	MEALS	BEFORE	AFTER	NOTES
TUES	Breakfast			
	Lunch			
	Supper			
	Snack			
	Bedtime			

DATE	MEALS	BEFORE	AFTER	NOTES
WED	Breakfast			
	Lunch			
	Supper			
	Snack			
	Bedtime			

DATE	MEALS	BEFORE	AFTER	NOTES
THUR	Breakfast			
	Lunch			
	Supper			
	Snack			
	Bedtime			

DATE	MEALS	BEFORE	AFTER	NOTES
FRI	Breakfast			
	Lunch			
	Supper			
	Snack			
	Bedtime			

DATE	MEALS	BEFORE	AFTER	NOTES
SAT	Breakfast			
	Lunch			
	Supper			
	Snack			
	Bedtime			

DATE	MEALS	BEFORE	AFTER	NOTES
SUN	Breakfast			
	Lunch			
	Supper			
	Snack			
	Bedtime			

DATE	MEALS	BEFORE	AFTER	NOTES
MON	Breakfast			
	Lunch			
	Supper			
	Snack			
	Bedtime			

DATE	MEALS	BEFORE	AFTER	NOTES
TUES	Breakfast			
	Lunch			
	Supper			
	Snack			
	Bedtime			

DATE	MEALS	BEFORE	AFTER	NOTES
WED	Breakfast			
	Lunch			
	Supper			
	Snack			
	Bedtime			

DATE	MEALS	BEFORE	AFTER	NOTES
THUR	Breakfast			
	Lunch			
	Supper			
	Snack			
	Bedtime			

DATE	MEALS	BEFORE	AFTER	NOTES
FRI	Breakfast			
	Lunch			
	Supper			
	Snack			
	Bedtime			

DATE	MEALS	BEFORE	AFTER	NOTES
SAT	Breakfast			
	Lunch			
	Supper			
	Snack			
	Bedtime			

DATE	MEALS	BEFORE	AFTER	NOTES
SUN	Breakfast			
	Lunch			
	Supper			
	Snack			
	Bedtime			

DATE	MEALS	BEFORE	AFTER	NOTES
MON	Breakfast			
	Lunch			
	Supper			
	Snack			
	Bedtime			

DATE	MEALS	BEFORE	AFTER	NOTES
TUES	Breakfast			
	Lunch			
	Supper			
	Snack			
	Bedtime			

DATE	MEALS	BEFORE	AFTER	NOTES
WED	Breakfast			
	Lunch			
	Supper			
	Snack			
	Bedtime			

DATE	MEALS	BEFORE	AFTER	NOTES
THUR	Breakfast			
	Lunch			
	Supper			
	Snack			
	Bedtime			

DATE	MEALS	BEFORE	AFTER	NOTES
FRI	Breakfast			
	Lunch			
	Supper			
	Snack			
	Bedtime			

DATE	MEALS	BEFORE	AFTER	NOTES
SAT	Breakfast			
	Lunch			
	Supper			
	Snack			
	Bedtime			

DATE	MEALS	BEFORE	AFTER	NOTES
SUN	Breakfast			
	Lunch			
	Supper			
	Snack			
	Bedtime			

DATE	MEALS	BEFORE	AFTER	NOTES
MON	Breakfast			
	Lunch			
	Supper			
	Snack			
	Bedtime			

DATE	MEALS	BEFORE	AFTER	NOTES
TUES	Breakfast			
	Lunch			
	Supper			
	Snack			
	Bedtime			

DATE	MEALS	BEFORE	AFTER	NOTES
WED	Breakfast			
	Lunch			
	Supper			
	Snack			
	Bedtime			

DATE	MEALS	BEFORE	AFTER	NOTES
THUR	Breakfast			
	Lunch			
	Supper			
	Snack			
	Bedtime			

DATE	MEALS	BEFORE	AFTER	NOTES
FRI	Breakfast			
	Lunch			
	Supper			
	Snack			
	Bedtime			

DATE	MEALS	BEFORE	AFTER	NOTES
SAT	Breakfast			
	Lunch			
	Supper			
	Snack			
	Bedtime			

DATE	MEALS	BEFORE	AFTER	NOTES
SUN	Breakfast			
	Lunch			
	Supper			
	Snack			
	Bedtime			

DATE	MEALS	BEFORE	AFTER	NOTES
MON	Breakfast			
	Lunch			
	Supper			
	Snack			
	Bedtime			

DATE	MEALS	BEFORE	AFTER	NOTES
TUES	Breakfast			
	Lunch			
	Supper			
	Snack			
	Bedtime			

DATE	MEALS	BEFORE	AFTER	NOTES
WED	Breakfast			
	Lunch			
	Supper			
	Snack			
	Bedtime			

DATE	MEALS	BEFORE	AFTER	NOTES
THUR	Breakfast			
	Lunch			
	Supper			
	Snack			
	Bedtime			

DATE	MEALS	BEFORE	AFTER	NOTES
FRI	Breakfast			
	Lunch			
	Supper			
	Snack			
	Bedtime			

DATE	MEALS	BEFORE	AFTER	NOTES
SAT	Breakfast			
	Lunch			
	Supper			
	Snack			
	Bedtime			

DATE	MEALS	BEFORE	AFTER	NOTES
SUN	Breakfast			
	Lunch			
	Supper			
	Snack			
	Bedtime			

DATE	MEALS	BEFORE	AFTER	NOTES
MON	Breakfast			
	Lunch			
	Supper			
	Snack			
	Bedtime			

DATE	MEALS	BEFORE	AFTER	NOTES
TUES	Breakfast			
	Lunch			
	Supper			
	Snack			
	Bedtime			

DATE	MEALS	BEFORE	AFTER	NOTES
WED	Breakfast			
	Lunch			
	Supper			
	Snack			
	Bedtime			

DATE	MEALS	BEFORE	AFTER	NOTES
THUR	Breakfast			
	Lunch			
	Supper			
	Snack			
	Bedtime			

DATE	MEALS	BEFORE	AFTER	NOTES
FRI	Breakfast			
	Lunch			
	Supper			
	Snack			
	Bedtime			

DATE	MEALS	BEFORE	AFTER	NOTES
SAT	Breakfast			
	Lunch			
	Supper			
	Snack			
	Bedtime			

DATE	MEALS	BEFORE	AFTER	NOTES
SUN	Breakfast			
	Lunch			
	Supper			
	Snack			
	Bedtime			

DATE	MEALS	BEFORE	AFTER	NOTES
MON	Breakfast			
	Lunch			
	Supper			
	Snack			
	Bedtime			

DATE	MEALS	BEFORE	AFTER	NOTES
TUES	Breakfast			
	Lunch			
	Supper			
	Snack			
	Bedtime			

DATE	MEALS	BEFORE	AFTER	NOTES
WED	Breakfast			
	Lunch			
	Supper			
	Snack			
	Bedtime			

DATE	MEALS	BEFORE	AFTER	NOTES
THUR	Breakfast			
	Lunch			
	Supper			
	Snack			
	Bedtime			

DATE	MEALS	BEFORE	AFTER	NOTES
FRI	Breakfast			
	Lunch			
	Supper			
	Snack			
	Bedtime			

DATE	MEALS	BEFORE	AFTER	NOTES
SAT	Breakfast			
	Lunch			
	Supper			
	Snack			
	Bedtime			

DATE	MEALS	BEFORE	AFTER	NOTES
SUN	Breakfast			
	Lunch			
	Supper			
	Snack			
	Bedtime			

DATE	MEALS	BEFORE	AFTER	NOTES
MON	Breakfast			
	Lunch			
	Supper			
	Snack			
	Bedtime			

DATE	MEALS	BEFORE	AFTER	NOTES
TUES	Breakfast			
	Lunch			
	Supper			
	Snack			
	Bedtime			

DATE	MEALS	BEFORE	AFTER	NOTES
WED	Breakfast			
	Lunch			
	Supper			
	Snack			
	Bedtime			

DATE	MEALS	BEFORE	AFTER	NOTES
THUR	Breakfast			
	Lunch			
	Supper			
	Snack			
	Bedtime			

DATE	MEALS	BEFORE	AFTER	NOTES
FRI	Breakfast			
	Lunch			
	Supper			
	Snack			
	Bedtime			

DATE	MEALS	BEFORE	AFTER	NOTES
SAT	Breakfast			
	Lunch			
	Supper			
	Snack			
	Bedtime			

DATE	MEALS	BEFORE	AFTER	NOTES
SUN	Breakfast			
	Lunch			
	Supper			
	Snack			
	Bedtime			

DATE	MEALS	BEFORE	AFTER	NOTES
MON	Breakfast			
	Lunch			
	Supper			
	Snack			
	Bedtime			

DATE	MEALS	BEFORE	AFTER	NOTES
TUES	Breakfast			
	Lunch			
	Supper			
	Snack			
	Bedtime			

DATE	MEALS	BEFORE	AFTER	NOTES
WED	Breakfast			
	Lunch			
	Supper			
	Snack			
	Bedtime			

DATE	MEALS	BEFORE	AFTER	NOTES
THUR	Breakfast			
	Lunch			
	Supper			
	Snack			
	Bedtime			

DATE	MEALS	BEFORE	AFTER	NOTES
FRI	Breakfast			
	Lunch			
	Supper			
	Snack			
	Bedtime			

DATE	MEALS	BEFORE	AFTER	NOTES
SAT	Breakfast			
	Lunch			
	Supper			
	Snack			
	Bedtime			

DATE	MEALS	BEFORE	AFTER	NOTES
SUN	Breakfast			
	Lunch			
	Supper			
	Snack			
	Bedtime			

DATE	MEALS	BEFORE	AFTER	NOTES
MON	Breakfast			
	Lunch			
	Supper			
	Snack			
	Bedtime			

DATE	MEALS	BEFORE	AFTER	NOTES
TUES	Breakfast			
	Lunch			
	Supper			
	Snack			
	Bedtime			

DATE	MEALS	BEFORE	AFTER	NOTES
WED	Breakfast			
	Lunch			
	Supper			
	Snack			
	Bedtime			

DATE	MEALS	BEFORE	AFTER	NOTES
THUR	Breakfast			
	Lunch			
	Supper			
	Snack			
	Bedtime			

DATE	MEALS	BEFORE	AFTER	NOTES
FRI	Breakfast			
	Lunch			
	Supper			
	Snack			
	Bedtime			

DATE	MEALS	BEFORE	AFTER	NOTES
SAT	Breakfast			
	Lunch			
	Supper			
	Snack			
	Bedtime			

DATE	MEALS	BEFORE	AFTER	NOTES
SUN	Breakfast			
	Lunch			
	Supper			
	Snack			
	Bedtime			

DATE	MEALS	BEFORE	AFTER	NOTES
MON	Breakfast			
	Lunch			
	Supper			
	Snack			
	Bedtime			

DATE	MEALS	BEFORE	AFTER	NOTES
TUES	Breakfast			
	Lunch			
	Supper			
	Snack			
	Bedtime			

DATE	MEALS	BEFORE	AFTER	NOTES
WED	Breakfast			
	Lunch			
	Supper			
	Snack			
	Bedtime			

DATE	MEALS	BEFORE	AFTER	NOTES
THUR	Breakfast			
	Lunch			
	Supper			
	Snack			
	Bedtime			

DATE	MEALS	BEFORE	AFTER	NOTES
FRI	Breakfast			
	Lunch			
	Supper			
	Snack			
	Bedtime			

DATE	MEALS	BEFORE	AFTER	NOTES
SAT	Breakfast			
	Lunch			
	Supper			
	Snack			
	Bedtime			

DATE	MEALS	BEFORE	AFTER	NOTES
SUN	Breakfast			
	Lunch			
	Supper			
	Snack			
	Bedtime			

DATE	MEALS	BEFORE	AFTER	NOTES
MON	Breakfast			
	Lunch			
	Supper			
	Snack			
	Bedtime			

DATE	MEALS	BEFORE	AFTER	NOTES
TUES	Breakfast			
	Lunch			
	Supper			
	Snack			
	Bedtime			

DATE	MEALS	BEFORE	AFTER	NOTES
WED	Breakfast			
	Lunch			
	Supper			
	Snack			
	Bedtime			

DATE	MEALS	BEFORE	AFTER	NOTES
THUR	Breakfast			
	Lunch			
	Supper			
	Snack			
	Bedtime			

DATE	MEALS	BEFORE	AFTER	NOTES
FRI	Breakfast			
	Lunch			
	Supper			
	Snack			
	Bedtime			

DATE	MEALS	BEFORE	AFTER	NOTES
SAT	Breakfast			
	Lunch			
	Supper			
	Snack			
	Bedtime			

DATE	MEALS	BEFORE	AFTER	NOTES
SUN	Breakfast			
	Lunch			
	Supper			
	Snack			
	Bedtime			

DATE	MEALS	BEFORE	AFTER	NOTES
MON	Breakfast			
	Lunch			
	Supper			
	Snack			
	Bedtime			

DATE	MEALS	BEFORE	AFTER	NOTES
TUES	Breakfast			
	Lunch			
	Supper			
	Snack			
	Bedtime			

DATE	MEALS	BEFORE	AFTER	NOTES
WED	Breakfast			
	Lunch			
	Supper			
	Snack			
	Bedtime			

DATE	MEALS	BEFORE	AFTER	NOTES
THUR	Breakfast			
	Lunch			
	Supper			
	Snack			
	Bedtime			

DATE	MEALS	BEFORE	AFTER	NOTES
FRI	Breakfast			
	Lunch			
	Supper			
	Snack			
	Bedtime			

DATE	MEALS	BEFORE	AFTER	NOTES
SAT	Breakfast			
	Lunch			
	Supper			
	Snack			
	Bedtime			

DATE	MEALS	BEFORE	AFTER	NOTES
SUN	Breakfast			
	Lunch			
	Supper			
	Snack			
	Bedtime			

DATE	MEALS	BEFORE	AFTER	NOTES
MON	Breakfast			
	Lunch			
	Supper			
	Snack			
	Bedtime			

DATE	MEALS	BEFORE	AFTER	NOTES
TUES	Breakfast			
	Lunch			
	Supper			
	Snack			
	Bedtime			

DATE	MEALS	BEFORE	AFTER	NOTES
WED	Breakfast			
	Lunch			
	Supper			
	Snack			
	Bedtime			

DATE	MEALS	BEFORE	AFTER	NOTES
THUR	Breakfast			
	Lunch			
	Supper			
	Snack			
	Bedtime			

DATE	MEALS	BEFORE	AFTER	NOTES
FRI	Breakfast			
	Lunch			
	Supper			
	Snack			
	Bedtime			

DATE	MEALS	BEFORE	AFTER	NOTES
SAT	Breakfast			
	Lunch			
	Supper			
	Snack			
	Bedtime			

DATE	MEALS	BEFORE	AFTER	NOTES
SUN	Breakfast			
	Lunch			
	Supper			
	Snack			
	Bedtime			

DATE	MEALS	BEFORE	AFTER	NOTES
MON	Breakfast			
	Lunch			
	Supper			
	Snack			
	Bedtime			

DATE	MEALS	BEFORE	AFTER	NOTES
TUES	Breakfast			
	Lunch			
	Supper			
	Snack			
	Bedtime			

DATE	MEALS	BEFORE	AFTER	NOTES
WED	Breakfast			
	Lunch			
	Supper			
	Snack			
	Bedtime			

DATE	MEALS	BEFORE	AFTER	NOTES
THUR	Breakfast			
	Lunch			
	Supper			
	Snack			
	Bedtime			

DATE	MEALS	BEFORE	AFTER	NOTES
FRI	Breakfast			
	Lunch			
	Supper			
	Snack			
	Bedtime			

DATE	MEALS	BEFORE	AFTER	NOTES
SAT	Breakfast			
	Lunch			
	Supper			
	Snack			
	Bedtime			

DATE	MEALS	BEFORE	AFTER	NOTES
SUN	Breakfast			
	Lunch			
	Supper			
	Snack			
	Bedtime			

DATE	MEALS	BEFORE	AFTER	NOTES
MON	Breakfast			
	Lunch			
	Supper			
	Snack			
	Bedtime			

DATE	MEALS	BEFORE	AFTER	NOTES
TUES	Breakfast			
	Lunch			
	Supper			
	Snack			
	Bedtime			

DATE	MEALS	BEFORE	AFTER	NOTES
WED	Breakfast			
	Lunch			
	Supper			
	Snack			
	Bedtime			

DATE	MEALS	BEFORE	AFTER	NOTES
THUR	Breakfast			
	Lunch			
	Supper			
	Snack			
	Bedtime			

DATE	MEALS	BEFORE	AFTER	NOTES
FRI	Breakfast			
	Lunch			
	Supper			
	Snack			
	Bedtime			

DATE	MEALS	BEFORE	AFTER	NOTES
SAT	Breakfast			
	Lunch			
	Supper			
	Snack			
	Bedtime			

DATE	MEALS	BEFORE	AFTER	NOTES
SUN	Breakfast			
	Lunch			
	Supper			
	Snack			
	Bedtime			

DATE	MEALS	BEFORE	AFTER	NOTES
MON	Breakfast			
	Lunch			
	Supper			
	Snack			
	Bedtime			

DATE	MEALS	BEFORE	AFTER	NOTES
TUES	Breakfast			
	Lunch			
	Supper			
	Snack			
	Bedtime			

DATE	MEALS	BEFORE	AFTER	NOTES
WED	Breakfast			
	Lunch			
	Supper			
	Snack			
	Bedtime			

DATE	MEALS	BEFORE	AFTER	NOTES
THUR	Breakfast			
	Lunch			
	Supper			
	Snack			
	Bedtime			

DATE	MEALS	BEFORE	AFTER	NOTES
FRI	Breakfast			
	Lunch			
	Supper			
	Snack			
	Bedtime			

DATE	MEALS	BEFORE	AFTER	NOTES
SAT	Breakfast			
	Lunch			
	Supper			
	Snack			
	Bedtime			

DATE	MEALS	BEFORE	AFTER	NOTES
SUN	Breakfast			
	Lunch			
	Supper			
	Snack			
	Bedtime			

DATE	MEALS	BEFORE	AFTER	NOTES
MON	Breakfast			
	Lunch			
	Supper			
	Snack			
	Bedtime			

DATE	MEALS	BEFORE	AFTER	NOTES
TUES	Breakfast			
	Lunch			
	Supper			
	Snack			
	Bedtime			

DATE	MEALS	BEFORE	AFTER	NOTES
WED	Breakfast			
	Lunch			
	Supper			
	Snack			
	Bedtime			

DATE	MEALS	BEFORE	AFTER	NOTES
THUR	Breakfast			
	Lunch			
	Supper			
	Snack			
	Bedtime			

DATE	MEALS	BEFORE	AFTER	NOTES
FRI	Breakfast			
	Lunch			
	Supper			
	Snack			
	Bedtime			

DATE	MEALS	BEFORE	AFTER	NOTES
SAT	Breakfast			
	Lunch			
	Supper			
	Snack			
	Bedtime			

DATE	MEALS	BEFORE	AFTER	NOTES
SUN	Breakfast			
	Lunch			
	Supper			
	Snack			
	Bedtime			

DATE	MEALS	BEFORE	AFTER	NOTES
MON	Breakfast			
	Lunch			
	Supper			
	Snack			
	Bedtime			

DATE	MEALS	BEFORE	AFTER	NOTES
TUES	Breakfast			
	Lunch			
	Supper			
	Snack			
	Bedtime			

DATE	MEALS	BEFORE	AFTER	NOTES
WED	Breakfast			
	Lunch			
	Supper			
	Snack			
	Bedtime			

DATE	MEALS	BEFORE	AFTER	NOTES
THUR	Breakfast			
	Lunch			
	Supper			
	Snack			
	Bedtime			

DATE	MEALS	BEFORE	AFTER	NOTES
FRI	Breakfast			
	Lunch			
	Supper			
	Snack			
	Bedtime			

DATE	MEALS	BEFORE	AFTER	NOTES
SAT	Breakfast			
	Lunch			
	Supper			
	Snack			
	Bedtime			

DATE	MEALS	BEFORE	AFTER	NOTES
SUN	Breakfast			
	Lunch			
	Supper			
	Snack			
	Bedtime			

DATE	MEALS	BEFORE	AFTER	NOTES
MON	Breakfast			
	Lunch			
	Supper			
	Snack			
	Bedtime			

DATE	MEALS	BEFORE	AFTER	NOTES
TUES	Breakfast			
	Lunch			
	Supper			
	Snack			
	Bedtime			

DATE	MEALS	BEFORE	AFTER	NOTES
WED	Breakfast			
	Lunch			
	Supper			
	Snack			
	Bedtime			

DATE	MEALS	BEFORE	AFTER	NOTES
THUR	Breakfast			
	Lunch			
	Supper			
	Snack			
	Bedtime			

DATE	MEALS	BEFORE	AFTER	NOTES
FRI	Breakfast			
	Lunch			
	Supper			
	Snack			
	Bedtime			

DATE	MEALS	BEFORE	AFTER	NOTES
SAT	Breakfast			
	Lunch			
	Supper			
	Snack			
	Bedtime			

DATE	MEALS	BEFORE	AFTER	NOTES
SUN	Breakfast			
	Lunch			
	Supper			
	Snack			
	Bedtime			

DATE	MEALS	BEFORE	AFTER	NOTES
MON	Breakfast			
	Lunch			
	Supper			
	Snack			
	Bedtime			

DATE	MEALS	BEFORE	AFTER	NOTES
TUES	Breakfast			
	Lunch			
	Supper			
	Snack			
	Bedtime			

DATE	MEALS	BEFORE	AFTER	NOTES
WED	Breakfast			
	Lunch			
	Supper			
	Snack			
	Bedtime			

DATE	MEALS	BEFORE	AFTER	NOTES
THUR	Breakfast			
	Lunch			
	Supper			
	Snack			
	Bedtime			

DATE	MEALS	BEFORE	AFTER	NOTES
FRI	Breakfast			
	Lunch			
	Supper			
	Snack			
	Bedtime			

DATE	MEALS	BEFORE	AFTER	NOTES
SAT	Breakfast			
	Lunch			
	Supper			
	Snack			
	Bedtime			

DATE	MEALS	BEFORE	AFTER	NOTES
SUN	Breakfast			
	Lunch			
	Supper			
	Snack			
	Bedtime			

DATE	MEALS	BEFORE	AFTER	NOTES
MON	Breakfast			
	Lunch			
	Supper			
	Snack			
	Bedtime			

DATE	MEALS	BEFORE	AFTER	NOTES
TUES	Breakfast			
	Lunch			
	Supper			
	Snack			
	Bedtime			

DATE	MEALS	BEFORE	AFTER	NOTES
WED	Breakfast			
	Lunch			
	Supper			
	Snack			
	Bedtime			

DATE	MEALS	BEFORE	AFTER	NOTES
THUR	Breakfast			
	Lunch			
	Supper			
	Snack			
	Bedtime			

DATE	MEALS	BEFORE	AFTER	NOTES
FRI	Breakfast			
	Lunch			
	Supper			
	Snack			
	Bedtime			

DATE	MEALS	BEFORE	AFTER	NOTES
SAT	Breakfast			
	Lunch			
	Supper			
	Snack			
	Bedtime			

DATE	MEALS	BEFORE	AFTER	NOTES
SUN	Breakfast			
	Lunch			
	Supper			
	Snack			
	Bedtime			

DATE	MEALS	BEFORE	AFTER	NOTES
MON	Breakfast			
	Lunch			
	Supper			
	Snack			
	Bedtime			

DATE	MEALS	BEFORE	AFTER	NOTES
TUES	Breakfast			
	Lunch			
	Supper			
	Snack			
	Bedtime			

DATE	MEALS	BEFORE	AFTER	NOTES
WED	Breakfast			
	Lunch			
	Supper			
	Snack			
	Bedtime			

DATE	MEALS	BEFORE	AFTER	NOTES
THUR	Breakfast			
	Lunch			
	Supper			
	Snack			
	Bedtime			

DATE	MEALS	BEFORE	AFTER	NOTES
FRI	Breakfast			
	Lunch			
	Supper			
	Snack			
	Bedtime			

DATE	MEALS	BEFORE	AFTER	NOTES
SAT	Breakfast			
	Lunch			
	Supper			
	Snack			
	Bedtime			

DATE	MEALS	BEFORE	AFTER	NOTES
SUN	Breakfast			
	Lunch			
	Supper			
	Snack			
	Bedtime			

DATE	MEALS	BEFORE	AFTER	NOTES
MON	Breakfast			
	Lunch			
	Supper			
	Snack			
	Bedtime			

DATE	MEALS	BEFORE	AFTER	NOTES
TUES	Breakfast			
	Lunch			
	Supper			
	Snack			
	Bedtime			

DATE	MEALS	BEFORE	AFTER	NOTES
WED	Breakfast			
	Lunch			
	Supper			
	Snack			
	Bedtime			

DATE	MEALS	BEFORE	AFTER	NOTES
THUR	Breakfast			
	Lunch			
	Supper			
	Snack			
	Bedtime			

DATE	MEALS	BEFORE	AFTER	NOTES
FRI	Breakfast			
	Lunch			
	Supper			
	Snack			
	Bedtime			

DATE	MEALS	BEFORE	AFTER	NOTES
SAT	Breakfast			
	Lunch			
	Supper			
	Snack			
	Bedtime			

DATE	MEALS	BEFORE	AFTER	NOTES
SUN	Breakfast			
	Lunch			
	Supper			
	Snack			
	Bedtime			

DATE	MEALS	BEFORE	AFTER	NOTES
MON	Breakfast			
	Lunch			
	Supper			
	Snack			
	Bedtime			

DATE	MEALS	BEFORE	AFTER	NOTES
TUES	Breakfast			
	Lunch			
	Supper			
	Snack			
	Bedtime			

DATE	MEALS	BEFORE	AFTER	NOTES
WED	Breakfast			
	Lunch			
	Supper			
	Snack			
	Bedtime			

DATE	MEALS	BEFORE	AFTER	NOTES
THUR	Breakfast			
	Lunch			
	Supper			
	Snack			
	Bedtime			

DATE	MEALS	BEFORE	AFTER	NOTES
FRI	Breakfast			
	Lunch			
	Supper			
	Snack			
	Bedtime			

DATE	MEALS	BEFORE	AFTER	NOTES
SAT	Breakfast			
	Lunch			
	Supper			
	Snack			
	Bedtime			

DATE	MEALS	BEFORE	AFTER	NOTES
SUN	Breakfast			
	Lunch			
	Supper			
	Snack			
	Bedtime			

DATE	MEALS	BEFORE	AFTER	NOTES
MON	Breakfast			
	Lunch			
	Supper			
	Snack			
	Bedtime			

DATE	MEALS	BEFORE	AFTER	NOTES
TUES	Breakfast			
	Lunch			
	Supper			
	Snack			
	Bedtime			

DATE	MEALS	BEFORE	AFTER	NOTES
WED	Breakfast			
	Lunch			
	Supper			
	Snack			
	Bedtime			

DATE	MEALS	BEFORE	AFTER	NOTES
THUR	Breakfast			
	Lunch			
	Supper			
	Snack			
	Bedtime			

DATE	MEALS	BEFORE	AFTER	NOTES
FRI	Breakfast			
	Lunch			
	Supper			
	Snack			
	Bedtime			

DATE	MEALS	BEFORE	AFTER	NOTES
SAT	Breakfast			
	Lunch			
	Supper			
	Snack			
	Bedtime			

DATE	MEALS	BEFORE	AFTER	NOTES
SUN	Breakfast			
	Lunch			
	Supper			
	Snack			
	Bedtime			

DATE	MEALS	BEFORE	AFTER	NOTES
MON	Breakfast			
	Lunch			
	Supper			
	Snack			
	Bedtime			

DATE	MEALS	BEFORE	AFTER	NOTES
TUES	Breakfast			
	Lunch			
	Supper			
	Snack			
	Bedtime			

DATE	MEALS	BEFORE	AFTER	NOTES
WED	Breakfast			
	Lunch			
	Supper			
	Snack			
	Bedtime			

DATE	MEALS	BEFORE	AFTER	NOTES
THUR	Breakfast			
	Lunch			
	Supper			
	Snack			
	Bedtime			

DATE	MEALS	BEFORE	AFTER	NOTES
FRI	Breakfast			
	Lunch			
	Supper			
	Snack			
	Bedtime			

DATE	MEALS	BEFORE	AFTER	NOTES
SAT	Breakfast			
	Lunch			
	Supper			
	Snack			
	Bedtime			

DATE	MEALS	BEFORE	AFTER	NOTES
SUN	Breakfast			
	Lunch			
	Supper			
	Snack			
	Bedtime			

DATE	MEALS	BEFORE	AFTER	NOTES
MON	Breakfast			
	Lunch			
	Supper			
	Snack			
	Bedtime			

DATE	MEALS	BEFORE	AFTER	NOTES
TUES	Breakfast			
	Lunch			
	Supper			
	Snack			
	Bedtime			

DATE	MEALS	BEFORE	AFTER	NOTES
WED	Breakfast			
	Lunch			
	Supper			
	Snack			
	Bedtime			

DATE	MEALS	BEFORE	AFTER	NOTES
THUR	Breakfast			
	Lunch			
	Supper			
	Snack			
	Bedtime			

DATE	MEALS	BEFORE	AFTER	NOTES
FRI	Breakfast			
	Lunch			
	Supper			
	Snack			
	Bedtime			

DATE	MEALS	BEFORE	AFTER	NOTES
SAT	Breakfast			
	Lunch			
	Supper			
	Snack			
	Bedtime			

DATE	MEALS	BEFORE	AFTER	NOTES
SUN	Breakfast			
	Lunch			
	Supper			
	Snack			
	Bedtime			

DATE	MEALS	BEFORE	AFTER	NOTES
MON	Breakfast			
	Lunch			
	Supper			
	Snack			
	Bedtime			

DATE	MEALS	BEFORE	AFTER	NOTES
TUES	Breakfast			
	Lunch			
	Supper			
	Snack			
	Bedtime			

DATE	MEALS	BEFORE	AFTER	NOTES
WED	Breakfast			
	Lunch			
	Supper			
	Snack			
	Bedtime			

DATE	MEALS	BEFORE	AFTER	NOTES
THUR	Breakfast			
	Lunch			
	Supper			
	Snack			
	Bedtime			

DATE	MEALS	BEFORE	AFTER	NOTES
FRI	Breakfast			
	Lunch			
	Supper			
	Snack			
	Bedtime			

DATE	MEALS	BEFORE	AFTER	NOTES
SAT	Breakfast			
	Lunch			
	Supper			
	Snack			
	Bedtime			

DATE	MEALS	BEFORE	AFTER	NOTES
SUN	Breakfast			
	Lunch			
	Supper			
	Snack			
	Bedtime			

DATE	MEALS	BEFORE	AFTER	NOTES
MON	Breakfast			
	Lunch			
	Supper			
	Snack			
	Bedtime			

DATE	MEALS	BEFORE	AFTER	NOTES
TUES	Breakfast			
	Lunch			
	Supper			
	Snack			
	Bedtime			

DATE	MEALS	BEFORE	AFTER	NOTES
WED	Breakfast			
	Lunch			
	Supper			
	Snack			
	Bedtime			

DATE	MEALS	BEFORE	AFTER	NOTES
THUR	Breakfast			
	Lunch			
	Supper			
	Snack			
	Bedtime			

DATE	MEALS	BEFORE	AFTER	NOTES
FRI	Breakfast			
	Lunch			
	Supper			
	Snack			
	Bedtime			

DATE	MEALS	BEFORE	AFTER	NOTES
SAT	Breakfast			
	Lunch			
	Supper			
	Snack			
	Bedtime			

DATE	MEALS	BEFORE	AFTER	NOTES
SUN	Breakfast			
	Lunch			
	Supper			
	Snack			
	Bedtime			

DATE	MEALS	BEFORE	AFTER	NOTES
MON	Breakfast			
	Lunch			
	Supper			
	Snack			
	Bedtime			

DATE	MEALS	BEFORE	AFTER	NOTES
TUES	Breakfast			
	Lunch			
	Supper			
	Snack			
	Bedtime			

DATE	MEALS	BEFORE	AFTER	NOTES
WED	Breakfast			
	Lunch			
	Supper			
	Snack			
	Bedtime			

DATE	MEALS	BEFORE	AFTER	NOTES
THUR	Breakfast			
	Lunch			
	Supper			
	Snack			
	Bedtime			

DATE	MEALS	BEFORE	AFTER	NOTES
FRI	Breakfast			
	Lunch			
	Supper			
	Snack			
	Bedtime			

DATE	MEALS	BEFORE	AFTER	NOTES
SAT	Breakfast			
	Lunch			
	Supper			
	Snack			
	Bedtime			

DATE	MEALS	BEFORE	AFTER	NOTES
SUN	Breakfast			
	Lunch			
	Supper			
	Snack			
	Bedtime			

DATE	MEALS	BEFORE	AFTER	NOTES
MON	Breakfast			
	Lunch			
	Supper			
	Snack			
	Bedtime			

DATE	MEALS	BEFORE	AFTER	NOTES
TUES	Breakfast			
	Lunch			
	Supper			
	Snack			
	Bedtime			

DATE	MEALS	BEFORE	AFTER	NOTES
WED	Breakfast			
	Lunch			
	Supper			
	Snack			
	Bedtime			

DATE	MEALS	BEFORE	AFTER	NOTES
THUR	Breakfast			
	Lunch			
	Supper			
	Snack			
	Bedtime			

DATE	MEALS	BEFORE	AFTER	NOTES
FRI	Breakfast			
	Lunch			
	Supper			
	Snack			
	Bedtime			

DATE	MEALS	BEFORE	AFTER	NOTES
SAT	Breakfast			
	Lunch			
	Supper			
	Snack			
	Bedtime			

DATE	MEALS	BEFORE	AFTER	NOTES
SUN	Breakfast			
	Lunch			
	Supper			
	Snack			
	Bedtime			

DATE	MEALS	BEFORE	AFTER	NOTES
MON	Breakfast			
	Lunch			
	Supper			
	Snack			
	Bedtime			

DATE	MEALS	BEFORE	AFTER	NOTES
TUES	Breakfast			
	Lunch			
	Supper			
	Snack			
	Bedtime			

DATE	MEALS	BEFORE	AFTER	NOTES
WED	Breakfast			
	Lunch			
	Supper			
	Snack			
	Bedtime			

DATE	MEALS	BEFORE	AFTER	NOTES
THUR	Breakfast			
	Lunch			
	Supper			
	Snack			
	Bedtime			

DATE	MEALS	BEFORE	AFTER	NOTES
FRI	Breakfast			
	Lunch			
	Supper			
	Snack			
	Bedtime			

DATE	MEALS	BEFORE	AFTER	NOTES
SAT	Breakfast			
	Lunch			
	Supper			
	Snack			
	Bedtime			

DATE	MEALS	BEFORE	AFTER	NOTES
SUN	Breakfast			
	Lunch			
	Supper			
	Snack			
	Bedtime			

DATE	MEALS	BEFORE	AFTER	NOTES
MON	Breakfast			
	Lunch			
	Supper			
	Snack			
	Bedtime			

DATE	MEALS	BEFORE	AFTER	NOTES
TUES	Breakfast			
	Lunch			
	Supper			
	Snack			
	Bedtime			

DATE	MEALS	BEFORE	AFTER	NOTES
WED	Breakfast			
	Lunch			
	Supper			
	Snack			
	Bedtime			

DATE	MEALS	BEFORE	AFTER	NOTES
THUR	Breakfast			
	Lunch			
	Supper			
	Snack			
	Bedtime			

DATE	MEALS	BEFORE	AFTER	NOTES
FRI	Breakfast			
	Lunch			
	Supper			
	Snack			
	Bedtime			

DATE	MEALS	BEFORE	AFTER	NOTES
SAT	Breakfast			
	Lunch			
	Supper			
	Snack			
	Bedtime			

DATE	MEALS	BEFORE	AFTER	NOTES
SUN	Breakfast			
	Lunch			
	Supper			
	Snack			
	Bedtime			

DATE	MEALS	BEFORE	AFTER	NOTES
MON	Breakfast			
	Lunch			
	Supper			
	Snack			
	Bedtime			

DATE	MEALS	BEFORE	AFTER	NOTES
TUES	Breakfast			
	Lunch			
	Supper			
	Snack			
	Bedtime			

DATE	MEALS	BEFORE	AFTER	NOTES
WED	Breakfast			
	Lunch			
	Supper			
	Snack			
	Bedtime			

DATE	MEALS	BEFORE	AFTER	NOTES
THUR	Breakfast			
	Lunch			
	Supper			
	Snack			
	Bedtime			

DATE	MEALS	BEFORE	AFTER	NOTES
FRI	Breakfast			
	Lunch			
	Supper			
	Snack			
	Bedtime			

DATE	MEALS	BEFORE	AFTER	NOTES
SAT	Breakfast			
	Lunch			
	Supper			
	Snack			
	Bedtime			

DATE	MEALS	BEFORE	AFTER	NOTES
SUN	Breakfast			
	Lunch			
	Supper			
	Snack			
	Bedtime			

DATE	MEALS	BEFORE	AFTER	NOTES
MON	Breakfast			
	Lunch			
	Supper			
	Snack			
	Bedtime			

DATE	MEALS	BEFORE	AFTER	NOTES
TUES	Breakfast			
	Lunch			
	Supper			
	Snack			
	Bedtime			

DATE	MEALS	BEFORE	AFTER	NOTES
WED	Breakfast			
	Lunch			
	Supper			
	Snack			
	Bedtime			

DATE	MEALS	BEFORE	AFTER	NOTES
THUR	Breakfast			
	Lunch			
	Supper			
	Snack			
	Bedtime			

DATE	MEALS	BEFORE	AFTER	NOTES
FRI	Breakfast			
	Lunch			
	Supper			
	Snack			
	Bedtime			

DATE	MEALS	BEFORE	AFTER	NOTES
SAT	Breakfast			
	Lunch			
	Supper			
	Snack			
	Bedtime			

DATE	MEALS	BEFORE	AFTER	NOTES
SUN	Breakfast			
	Lunch			
	Supper			
	Snack			
	Bedtime			

DATE	MEALS	BEFORE	AFTER	NOTES
MON	Breakfast			
	Lunch			
	Supper			
	Snack			
	Bedtime			

DATE	MEALS	BEFORE	AFTER	NOTES
TUES	Breakfast			
	Lunch			
	Supper			
	Snack			
	Bedtime			

DATE	MEALS	BEFORE	AFTER	NOTES
WED	Breakfast			
	Lunch			
	Supper			
	Snack			
	Bedtime			

DATE	MEALS	BEFORE	AFTER	NOTES
THUR	Breakfast			
	Lunch			
	Supper			
	Snack			
	Bedtime			

DATE	MEALS	BEFORE	AFTER	NOTES
FRI	Breakfast			
	Lunch			
	Supper			
	Snack			
	Bedtime			

DATE	MEALS	BEFORE	AFTER	NOTES
SAT	Breakfast			
	Lunch			
	Supper			
	Snack			
	Bedtime			

DATE	MEALS	BEFORE	AFTER	NOTES
SUN	Breakfast			
	Lunch			
	Supper			
	Snack			
	Bedtime			

DATE	MEALS	BEFORE	AFTER	NOTES
MON	Breakfast			
	Lunch			
	Supper			
	Snack			
	Bedtime			

DATE	MEALS	BEFORE	AFTER	NOTES
TUES	Breakfast			
	Lunch			
	Supper			
	Snack			
	Bedtime			

DATE	MEALS	BEFORE	AFTER	NOTES
WED	Breakfast			
	Lunch			
	Supper			
	Snack			
	Bedtime			

DATE	MEALS	BEFORE	AFTER	NOTES
THUR	Breakfast			
	Lunch			
	Supper			
	Snack			
	Bedtime			

DATE	MEALS	BEFORE	AFTER	NOTES
FRI	Breakfast			
	Lunch			
	Supper			
	Snack			
	Bedtime			

DATE	MEALS	BEFORE	AFTER	NOTES
SAT	Breakfast			
	Lunch			
	Supper			
	Snack			
	Bedtime			

DATE	MEALS	BEFORE	AFTER	NOTES
SUN	Breakfast			
	Lunch			
	Supper			
	Snack			
	Bedtime			

DATE	MEALS	BEFORE	AFTER	NOTES
MON	Breakfast			
	Lunch			
	Supper			
	Snack			
	Bedtime			

DATE	MEALS	BEFORE	AFTER	NOTES
TUES	Breakfast			
	Lunch			
	Supper			
	Snack			
	Bedtime			

DATE	MEALS	BEFORE	AFTER	NOTES
WED	Breakfast			
	Lunch			
	Supper			
	Snack			
	Bedtime			

DATE	MEALS	BEFORE	AFTER	NOTES
THUR	Breakfast			
	Lunch			
	Supper			
	Snack			
	Bedtime			

DATE	MEALS	BEFORE	AFTER	NOTES
FRI	Breakfast			
	Lunch			
	Supper			
	Snack			
	Bedtime			

DATE	MEALS	BEFORE	AFTER	NOTES
SAT	Breakfast			
	Lunch			
	Supper			
	Snack			
	Bedtime			

DATE	MEALS	BEFORE	AFTER	NOTES
SUN	Breakfast			
	Lunch			
	Supper			
	Snack			
	Bedtime			

DATE	MEALS	BEFORE	AFTER	NOTES
MON	Breakfast			
	Lunch			
	Supper			
	Snack			
	Bedtime			

DATE	MEALS	BEFORE	AFTER	NOTES
TUES	Breakfast			
	Lunch			
	Supper			
	Snack			
	Bedtime			

DATE	MEALS	BEFORE	AFTER	NOTES
WED	Breakfast			
	Lunch			
	Supper			
	Snack			
	Bedtime			

DATE	MEALS	BEFORE	AFTER	NOTES
THUR	Breakfast			
	Lunch			
	Supper			
	Snack			
	Bedtime			

DATE	MEALS	BEFORE	AFTER	NOTES
FRI	Breakfast			
	Lunch			
	Supper			
	Snack			
	Bedtime			

DATE	MEALS	BEFORE	AFTER	NOTES
SAT	Breakfast			
	Lunch			
	Supper			
	Snack			
	Bedtime			

DATE	MEALS	BEFORE	AFTER	NOTES
SUN	Breakfast			
	Lunch			
	Supper			
	Snack			
	Bedtime			

DATE	MEALS	BEFORE	AFTER	NOTES
MON	Breakfast			
	Lunch			
	Supper			
	Snack			
	Bedtime			

DATE	MEALS	BEFORE	AFTER	NOTES
TUES	Breakfast			
	Lunch			
	Supper			
	Snack			
	Bedtime			

DATE	MEALS	BEFORE	AFTER	NOTES
WED	Breakfast			
	Lunch			
	Supper			
	Snack			
	Bedtime			

DATE	MEALS	BEFORE	AFTER	NOTES
THUR	Breakfast			
	Lunch			
	Supper			
	Snack			
	Bedtime			

DATE	MEALS	BEFORE	AFTER	NOTES
FRI	Breakfast			
	Lunch			
	Supper			
	Snack			
	Bedtime			

DATE	MEALS	BEFORE	AFTER	NOTES
SAT	Breakfast			
	Lunch			
	Supper			
	Snack			
	Bedtime			

DATE	MEALS	BEFORE	AFTER	NOTES
SUN	Breakfast			
	Lunch			
	Supper			
	Snack			
	Bedtime			

DATE	MEALS	BEFORE	AFTER	NOTES
MON	Breakfast			
	Lunch			
	Supper			
	Snack			
	Bedtime			

DATE	MEALS	BEFORE	AFTER	NOTES
TUES	Breakfast			
	Lunch			
	Supper			
	Snack			
	Bedtime			

DATE	MEALS	BEFORE	AFTER	NOTES
WED	Breakfast			
	Lunch			
	Supper			
	Snack			
	Bedtime			

DATE	MEALS	BEFORE	AFTER	NOTES
THUR	Breakfast			
	Lunch			
	Supper			
	Snack			
	Bedtime			

DATE	MEALS	BEFORE	AFTER	NOTES
FRI	Breakfast			
	Lunch			
	Supper			
	Snack			
	Bedtime			

DATE	MEALS	BEFORE	AFTER	NOTES
SAT	Breakfast			
	Lunch			
	Supper			
	Snack			
	Bedtime			

DATE	MEALS	BEFORE	AFTER	NOTES
SUN	Breakfast			
	Lunch			
	Supper			
	Snack			
	Bedtime			

DATE	MEALS	BEFORE	AFTER	NOTES
MON	Breakfast			
	Lunch			
	Supper			
	Snack			
	Bedtime			

DATE	MEALS	BEFORE	AFTER	NOTES
TUES	Breakfast			
	Lunch			
	Supper			
	Snack			
	Bedtime			

DATE	MEALS	BEFORE	AFTER	NOTES
WED	Breakfast			
	Lunch			
	Supper			
	Snack			
	Bedtime			

DATE	MEALS	BEFORE	AFTER	NOTES
THUR	Breakfast			
	Lunch			
	Supper			
	Snack			
	Bedtime			

DATE	MEALS	BEFORE	AFTER	NOTES
FRI	Breakfast			
	Lunch			
	Supper			
	Snack			
	Bedtime			

DATE	MEALS	BEFORE	AFTER	NOTES
SAT	Breakfast			
	Lunch			
	Supper			
	Snack			
	Bedtime			

DATE	MEALS	BEFORE	AFTER	NOTES
SUN	Breakfast			
	Lunch			
	Supper			
	Snack			
	Bedtime			

DATE	MEALS	BEFORE	AFTER	NOTES
MON	Breakfast			
	Lunch			
	Supper			
	Snack			
	Bedtime			

DATE	MEALS	BEFORE	AFTER	NOTES
TUES	Breakfast			
	Lunch			
	Supper			
	Snack			
	Bedtime			

DATE	MEALS	BEFORE	AFTER	NOTES
WED	Breakfast			
	Lunch			
	Supper			
	Snack			
	Bedtime			

DATE	MEALS	BEFORE	AFTER	NOTES
THUR	Breakfast			
	Lunch			
	Supper			
	Snack			
	Bedtime			

DATE	MEALS	BEFORE	AFTER	NOTES
FRI	Breakfast			
	Lunch			
	Supper			
	Snack			
	Bedtime			

DATE	MEALS	BEFORE	AFTER	NOTES
SAT	Breakfast			
	Lunch			
	Supper			
	Snack			
	Bedtime			

DATE	MEALS	BEFORE	AFTER	NOTES
SUN	Breakfast			
	Lunch			
	Supper			
	Snack			
	Bedtime			

DATE	MEALS	BEFORE	AFTER	NOTES
MON	Breakfast			
	Lunch			
	Supper			
	Snack			
	Bedtime			

DATE	MEALS	BEFORE	AFTER	NOTES
TUES	Breakfast			
	Lunch			
	Supper			
	Snack			
	Bedtime			

DATE	MEALS	BEFORE	AFTER	NOTES
WED	Breakfast			
	Lunch			
	Supper			
	Snack			
	Bedtime			

DATE	MEALS	BEFORE	AFTER	NOTES
THUR	Breakfast			
	Lunch			
	Supper			
	Snack			
	Bedtime			

DATE	MEALS	BEFORE	AFTER	NOTES
FRI	Breakfast			
	Lunch			
	Supper			
	Snack			
	Bedtime			

DATE	MEALS	BEFORE	AFTER	NOTES
SAT	Breakfast			
	Lunch			
	Supper			
	Snack			
	Bedtime			

DATE	MEALS	BEFORE	AFTER	NOTES
SUN	Breakfast			
	Lunch			
	Supper			
	Snack			
	Bedtime			

DATE	MEALS	BEFORE	AFTER	NOTES
MON	Breakfast			
	Lunch			
	Supper			
	Snack			
	Bedtime			

DATE	MEALS	BEFORE	AFTER	NOTES
TUES	Breakfast			
	Lunch			
	Supper			
	Snack			
	Bedtime			

DATE	MEALS	BEFORE	AFTER	NOTES
WED	Breakfast			
	Lunch			
	Supper			
	Snack			
	Bedtime			

DATE	MEALS	BEFORE	AFTER	NOTES
THUR	Breakfast			
	Lunch			
	Supper			
	Snack			
	Bedtime			

DATE	MEALS	BEFORE	AFTER	NOTES
FRI	Breakfast			
	Lunch			
	Supper			
	Snack			
	Bedtime			

DATE	MEALS	BEFORE	AFTER	NOTES
SAT	Breakfast			
	Lunch			
	Supper			
	Snack			
	Bedtime			

DATE	MEALS	BEFORE	AFTER	NOTES
SUN	Breakfast			
	Lunch			
	Supper			
	Snack			
	Bedtime			

DATE	MEALS	BEFORE	AFTER	NOTES
MON	Breakfast			
	Lunch			
	Supper			
	Snack			
	Bedtime			

DATE	MEALS	BEFORE	AFTER	NOTES
TUES	Breakfast			
	Lunch			
	Supper			
	Snack			
	Bedtime			

DATE	MEALS	BEFORE	AFTER	NOTES
WED	Breakfast			
	Lunch			
	Supper			
	Snack			
	Bedtime			

DATE	MEALS	BEFORE	AFTER	NOTES
THUR	Breakfast			
	Lunch			
	Supper			
	Snack			
	Bedtime			

DATE	MEALS	BEFORE	AFTER	NOTES
FRI	Breakfast			
	Lunch			
	Supper			
	Snack			
	Bedtime			

DATE	MEALS	BEFORE	AFTER	NOTES
SAT	Breakfast			
	Lunch			
	Supper			
	Snack			
	Bedtime			

DATE	MEALS	BEFORE	AFTER	NOTES
SUN	Breakfast			
	Lunch			
	Supper			
	Snack			
	Bedtime			

DATE	MEALS	BEFORE	AFTER	NOTES
MON	Breakfast			
	Lunch			
	Supper			
	Snack			
	Bedtime			

DATE	MEALS	BEFORE	AFTER	NOTES
TUES	Breakfast			
	Lunch			
	Supper			
	Snack			
	Bedtime			

DATE	MEALS	BEFORE	AFTER	NOTES
WED	Breakfast			
	Lunch			
	Supper			
	Snack			
	Bedtime			

DATE	MEALS	BEFORE	AFTER	NOTES
THUR	Breakfast			
	Lunch			
	Supper			
	Snack			
	Bedtime			

DATE	MEALS	BEFORE	AFTER	NOTES
FRI	Breakfast			
	Lunch			
	Supper			
	Snack			
	Bedtime			

DATE	MEALS	BEFORE	AFTER	NOTES
SAT	Breakfast			
	Lunch			
	Supper			
	Snack			
	Bedtime			

DATE	MEALS	BEFORE	AFTER	NOTES
SUN	Breakfast			
	Lunch			
	Supper			
	Snack			
	Bedtime			

DATE	MEALS	BEFORE	AFTER	NOTES
MON	Breakfast			
	Lunch			
	Supper			
	Snack			
	Bedtime			

DATE	MEALS	BEFORE	AFTER	NOTES
TUES	Breakfast			
	Lunch			
	Supper			
	Snack			
	Bedtime			

DATE	MEALS	BEFORE	AFTER	NOTES
WED	Breakfast			
	Lunch			
	Supper			
	Snack			
	Bedtime			

DATE	MEALS	BEFORE	AFTER	NOTES
THUR	Breakfast			
	Lunch			
	Supper			
	Snack			
	Bedtime			

DATE	MEALS	BEFORE	AFTER	NOTES
FRI	Breakfast			
	Lunch			
	Supper			
	Snack			
	Bedtime			

DATE	MEALS	BEFORE	AFTER	NOTES
SAT	Breakfast			
	Lunch			
	Supper			
	Snack			
	Bedtime			

DATE	MEALS	BEFORE	AFTER	NOTES
SUN	Breakfast			
	Lunch			
	Supper			
	Snack			
	Bedtime			

DATE	MEALS	BEFORE	AFTER	NOTES
MON	Breakfast			
	Lunch			
	Supper			
	Snack			
	Bedtime			

DATE	MEALS	BEFORE	AFTER	NOTES
TUES	Breakfast			
	Lunch			
	Supper			
	Snack			
	Bedtime			

DATE	MEALS	BEFORE	AFTER	NOTES
WED	Breakfast			
	Lunch			
	Supper			
	Snack			
	Bedtime			

DATE	MEALS	BEFORE	AFTER	NOTES
THUR	Breakfast			
	Lunch			
	Supper			
	Snack			
	Bedtime			

DATE	MEALS	BEFORE	AFTER	NOTES
FRI	Breakfast			
	Lunch			
	Supper			
	Snack			
	Bedtime			

DATE	MEALS	BEFORE	AFTER	NOTES
SAT	Breakfast			
	Lunch			
	Supper			
	Snack			
	Bedtime			

DATE	MEALS	BEFORE	AFTER	NOTES
SUN	Breakfast			
	Lunch			
	Supper			
	Snack			
	Bedtime			

DATE	MEALS	BEFORE	AFTER	NOTES
MON	Breakfast			
	Lunch			
	Supper			
	Snack			
	Bedtime			

DATE	MEALS	BEFORE	AFTER	NOTES
TUES	Breakfast			
	Lunch			
	Supper			
	Snack			
	Bedtime			

DATE	MEALS	BEFORE	AFTER	NOTES
WED	Breakfast			
	Lunch			
	Supper			
	Snack			
	Bedtime			

DATE	MEALS	BEFORE	AFTER	NOTES
THUR	Breakfast			
	Lunch			
	Supper			
	Snack			
	Bedtime			

DATE	MEALS	BEFORE	AFTER	NOTES
FRI	Breakfast			
	Lunch			
	Supper			
	Snack			
	Bedtime			

DATE	MEALS	BEFORE	AFTER	NOTES
SAT	Breakfast			
	Lunch			
	Supper			
	Snack			
	Bedtime			

DATE	MEALS	BEFORE	AFTER	NOTES
SUN	Breakfast			
	Lunch			
	Supper			
	Snack			
	Bedtime			

DATE	MEALS	BEFORE	AFTER	NOTES
MON	Breakfast			
	Lunch			
	Supper			
	Snack			
	Bedtime			

DATE	MEALS	BEFORE	AFTER	NOTES
TUES	Breakfast			
	Lunch			
	Supper			
	Snack			
	Bedtime			

DATE	MEALS	BEFORE	AFTER	NOTES
WED	Breakfast			
	Lunch			
	Supper			
	Snack			
	Bedtime			

DATE	MEALS	BEFORE	AFTER	NOTES
THUR	Breakfast			
	Lunch			
	Supper			
	Snack			
	Bedtime			

DATE	MEALS	BEFORE	AFTER	NOTES
FRI	Breakfast			
	Lunch			
	Supper			
	Snack			
	Bedtime			

DATE	MEALS	BEFORE	AFTER	NOTES
SAT	Breakfast			
	Lunch			
	Supper			
	Snack			
	Bedtime			

www.ingramcontent.com/pod-product-compliance
Lightning Source LLC
Chambersburg PA
CBHW071721020426
42333CB00017B/2355
9781953557131